OutSmart
AGING

9 ANTI-AGING SECRETS
THAT WILL CHANGE YOUR LIFE

DR. KEVIN LIGHT

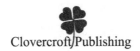
Clovercroft Publishing

OutSmart Aging: 9 Anti-Aging Secrets That Will Change Your Life

© 2014 by Dr. Kevin Light

Published by Clovercroft Publishing, Franklin, Tennessee

Concept Development by Tony Jeary

Edited by Tammy Kling

Cover Design by Debbie Manning Sheppard

Interior Layout Design by Suzanne Lawing

Copy Edit by Gail Fallen

Printed in the United States of America

978-1-940262-70-3

This first book is dedicated to my perfect wife, Dena, and my stellar family. Special thanks to the Lockhart family who graciously offered their beautiful home overlooking the mountains of Taos, New Mexico, where I spent weeks writing with inspiration under the Zia sun.

FOREWORD BY PHIL ROMANO

I've been an entrepreneur for years, and it's exciting, but it can be stressful. You have to find ways to manage your stress, no matter who you are or what you do. How do you look at life? Is your outlook positive or negative?

Life is an exciting adventure, but you only get one shot. I learned to be vigilant about living life full on after I was diagnosed with malignant lymphoma at age 50. I went through surgery and six months of chemotherapy. After that, I swore off all medications and started a healthy path. I was told to switch up my routine for both food and exercise, and I did. I not only started taking better care of myself; I actually began to listen to my doctor.

When I was diagnosed with cancer, I decided to be vigilant about living life as best as I could. Now is the time. Do it now! Live, love, laugh, and give back. I started a group called Hunger Busters, and we go out weekly and feed the homeless. It's a rewarding part of my life. I became involved in medical investments--both the stent, where I learned about cardiovascular disease, and the lap band, where I learned about obesity. I've invested in a lot of things, but the best investment I've ever made by far is in my own health.

I work out by walking, running, and lifting weights. Under the guidance of Dr. Light, I've now sharpened my focus on prevention, and I've developed a healthier routine. Health is my number one priority.

Is it yours? It should be. Without your health, there is no sense in having any other priorities, because you won't be around for long. Reading this book is a great commitment toward your health and wellness.

Aging and all of the new technologies surrounding the field of anti-aging are intriguing. There's so much you can do today to feel better—and look better, too. Turn the page, and apply some of these principles for youth to your own life. You'll be glad you did. Invest in your health—it's an investment well worth making.

PHIL ROMANO
Founder of Hunger Busters, Romano's Macaroni Grill, Fuddruckers, and Eatzi's . . . and father extraordinaire

INTRODUCTION

I've seen human hearts and other internal organs from the inside. I've held them in my hands and altered their structure when they were misbehaving. During surgery, I've had an up close and personal view of healthy versus unhealthy organs and have seen disease in full bloom. I've seen tired hearts, toxic lungs, and inflamed intestines. I know firsthand, inside and out, the ravages of chronic disease on the human species. I possess a peculiar perspective–an unusual vantage point that few physicians acquire. This isn't just theory. It's part of my reality.

As a general surgeon, I have operated on many different types of patients. The youngest was 5 days old. He had a heart condition, and I had to clip an abnormal connection between the aorta and the pulmonary artery in the neonatal intensive unit. I entered his tiny chest, and using powerful magnifying glasses, corrected nature's mistake—and he was fine. The oldest patient I ever worked on was 92, and I've done surgeries on everyone (and everything) in between. Smokers have lungs that are as black as tar. I've tried to sew damaged blood vessels together that were coated inside with rings of cholesterol-laden junk accumulated after years of poor choices in food and lifestyle. Some people I've worked on have organs encased in fat. It's hard to operate on them, because the fat is slippery and it makes the procedure more challenging and the recovery difficult. I've done belly surgery where I've literally had to cut down through twelve inches of fat, just to get to the internal organs. In surgery, we take the people who are critically Ill, whether they've lived a good lifestyle or not, and hope for the same outcome.

Life is lived in chapters, and I was compelled to leave the world of disease and illness to explore aesthetics and the impact of aging on the human form. As a cosmetic surgeon, I translated the surgical skills of preserving life to turning back the clock. And the clock ticks at different speeds for different people. The contrast in appearance between a 60-year-old woman who has lived a clean life out of the sun and a 32-year-old sun goddess smoker party-dog is astounding. Our skin tells our story–it reflects what may be lurking underneath. We can buff it up, laser it, and nip and tuck it. We can set back that clock–but it's like giving an old beat-up car a new paint job. It merely covers up what miles and miles of bad road have done to the inside.

I have taken the lessons learned from years of operating on sick people and offering the fountain of youth to aging people and applied them to the logical conclusion of this journey–Age Management Medicine. I have gone from fixing the consequences of aging to helping to slow the process down. Many people surrender to the inevitability of the aging process because of what they've read or have been taught; however, you truly are the architect of your own aging. Today my focus is on helping people discover that they are in control of their destinies: it simply comes down to personal choice.

My joy comes from waking people up and educating them by providing the tools to manage their aging. These tools include bioidentical hormone therapy, proper nutrition (avoiding high fat, high carb foods), essential supplementation, and fitness. And, even more than anything else, stress management.

Of all the weapons that blast away at us inside and out, stress is the most relentless and powerful. Whether it's physical, emotional, job-related, or financial, stress knocks our physiology off the tracks and drives poor lifestyle choices. Smoking, alcohol, and comfort food are what we grab to medicate stress. Poor sleep, lack of energy, and anxiety fogs up our brain and forces our physiology to burn fast and dirty. It beats us down and ushers in chronic disease and mental impairment.

If we want to preserve any reasonable quality of life, we need to burn the candle of life slow and clean. The good news? You are in complete control of your stress.

The time to start is now–before the horse has left the barn. It's so much easier to prevent chronic disease and accelerated aging than it is to treat it. The steps outlined in this book are a recipe for a healthy, vigorous life, free from the maladies that plague Western culture. It is never too late to start. All it takes is a little knowledge and a lot of commitment. Shed the surrender mentality of inevitability, and reach for the prize of restoration and preservation of our most valuable asset–good health. It's worth more than fame and fortune. Get it and keep it while you can.

KEVIN LIGHT, DO, MBA
Dallas, Texas
2014

ACKNOWLEDGMENTS

My journey from general and cosmetic surgery to integrative medicine was accidental. While getting my MBA from the University of Texas at Austin, I temporarily started helping out at a 'functional medicine clinic'. I had my doubts about this functional medicine stuff. In my world people were 'really sick' with afflictions like gunshot wounds, acute appendicitis or colon cancer. Functional medicine focused on more subtle issues like how is your concentration, how are you sleeping at night, why are you gaining weight, what can we do to spark up your libido, or how can we lessen your chances of developing cancer someday? The tools of their trade included things like bio-identical hormones, lifestyle modification, nutritional supplements and exercise. I had never been exposed to any of this and it all sounded kind of new-age shaky to me. In fact, I didn't know what I didn't know.

Within days I began to see how this medicine transformed lives. I saw how simple non-invasive interventions based on science took the *surrender* out of the aches and pains of getting older and replaced it with joyful anticipation and *expectation* of health and vitality. I drank the kool-aid, became a 'believer' and plunged into fellowship training through the American Academy of Anti-Aging Medicine. I credit the Age Management Medical Group, Gary Osborn RPh, Jim Hrncir RPh and Filomen Trindade MD for their part in rounding out my expertise in Integrative and Functional medicine.

I never really ever planned on writing a book. I wondered who would want to read anything I wrote? What could I possibly contribute? Enter Julie Silver, MD. – Chief Editor of Books at Harvard Health Publications and director of the annual 3 –

day Harvard course geared toward health care providers titled "Publishing Books, Memoirs and Other Creative Nonfiction". She insisted that everyone had a unique experience and knowledge base – that we ALL had a story to tell. Her course motivated me to write this book.

Tara Coles, MD was my objective sounding board. Dr. Mike Woo-Ming and his partner Chris Huish convinced me that publishing was not as scary as it sounds. Tony Jeary and Tammy Kling have helped publish scores of beginning authors, including several doctors, and their knowledge of the industry and publishing connections were lifesaving.

Of course, family both supports AND ages you! My wife Dena, kids and their spouses Alex Light, Thomas and Emma Strong, Kristen and Sam Springthorpe, Caeden and Landen Springthorp, Richelle Light, Trisha, Ben and Levi Pennington have all been important players leading to this book.

"You only live once, but if you do it right, once is enough."
—MAE WEST

"The doctor of the future will be oneself."
—ALBERT SCHWEITZER

"The best six doctors anywhere
And no one can deny it
Are sunshine, water, rest, and air
Exercise and diet.
These six will gladly you attend
If only you are willing
Your mind they'll ease
Your will they'll mend
And charge you not a shilling."

—NURSERY RHYME QUOTED BY WAYNE FIELDS,
WHAT THE RIVER KNOWS, 1990

CONTENTS

CHAPTER 1

WHY DO WE AGE?

One of the big problems in society today is the idea that aging is normal.

We have been led to believe that the emotional, cognitive, and physical decline that we experience as we age is an immutable fact of life like the sunrise and taxes. It is a "surrender" mentality based on myth and not knowing any better.

So here's how it looks: "Yes, I know I should eat better and exercise and quit smoking and try not to get so stressed out, but, hey: we all have to die sometime." But tons of research clearly demonstrates that our rate of aging can be influenced and altered significantly. In fact, aging is largely a result of our choices, our lifestyle, versus a predetermined genetic "plan" that we robotically follow like a computer reading software. In reality, how you age is largely up to you!

You can be old, fat, and sick at 60 or youthful, fit and vibrant.

The choice is yours.

In a perfect world, we would all hum along living relatively healthy lives. Then when our "time" comes, we'd just check out. Instead of having a gradual decline in our health after our 50th birthday, it would be nice if we could "square off" our life curve and just leave the party when our warranty wore out. The good news is that several lifestyle changes and easy interventions can go a long way in achieving a healthy mind, body, and spirit as we blast past the 50s, 60s, 70s, 80s--and even the 90s.

WHAT IS AGING?

Physiologically we peak in our 20s, start to falloff in our 30s, and begin our sharp decline in our 40s. Then aging really takes off. On average, in the United States during the ten-year span between the ages of 40 and 50, men will age physiologically 15.2 years and women will age 18.6 years.

As individuals, we will age at variable rates due to our genetic predispositions and chosen lifestyles involving the quality of our diet, activity level, bad habits such as smoking and excessive alcohol consumption, and the subsequent onset of diseases such as high blood pressure, obesity, and diabetes.

SO WHAT HAPPENS?

- Our brain shrinks and there is loss of cognitive function and focus and memory.
- Our hearing becomes impaired, primarily for higher pitches.
- Our vision starts to fall apart with loss of visual acuity, color perception, and the development of imperfections in the lens of our eye, called cataracts.
- We start lose our sense of taste and smell.
- We lose collagen and elasticity in our skin causing it to be

thin and wrinkly, heal poorly, and bruise easily. Age spots dot our skin like an Appaloosa's, connective tissues stretch, and body parts (butts, faces, arms, tummy, and breasts) start to sag.

- We lose muscle and bone and gain fat, resulting in less strength, osteoporosis, and the onset of obesity.
- Our organs, such as our heart, lungs, kidneys, and pancreas, start to feel the effects of years of use and abuse and can no longer "keep their head above water" and start their long slide toward failure.
- The output of hormones from our glands drop, either because the glands themselves fail, or the brain does not "drive" them properly anymore. This adversely affects every single cell in our body.

But can we reverse this process? Let's look at why and how we age.

THE PHYSICS OF AGING?

The common denominator of all aging theories is the tendency for complex biological systems to naturally lose energy and "fall apart." This has something to do with the second law of thermodynamics, which basically says that anything in the universe with a system or structure naturally tends to disintegrate when left to its own devices. Our wonderful physiology circumvents this inevitability with several complex repair systems. This repair system is generally rocking and rolling until our late 20s and early 30s. It then starts to slowly splutter and backfire. As we enter our early 40s, our repair systems fall prey themselves to the second law of thermodynamics: now our *repair systems need repair*, and the changes known as aging begin to manifest with a vengeance.

From a species-survival perspective, our carefully engineered biology is designed to balance the physiologic disruption and repair equation in favor of repair, at least until reproductive maturity. However, after we blaze through reproductive maturity, our repair systems become "out of warranty," and we start hitting speed bumps as we continue our journey through life. And, depending upon how brightly and intensely we burned our candle in our earlier years, our aging experience ranges from subtle (think Doogie Howser) to severe (look at the face of any former president of the United States).

THE THEORIES OF AGING

At the cellular level, several little housekeeping chores don't get done, and our clean, pristine, perfect cells start to crumble, sputter, and misfire. Author and scientist Dr. de Grey defines aging as "the effect of accumulated side effects from our metabolism that eventually kills us. de Grey is famous for his articles on the seven causes of aging. They include:

Accumulation of junk outside of our cells—This is the junk yard of the cells, where they throw away their trash. It keeps getting bigger over time. This is a big problem in the brain (Alzheimer's disease).

Accumulation of junk inside of our cells—Biological waste products can build up inside the cells as well, especially with prolonged exposure to toxins (tobacco) and stress (inflammation). This is a huge problem for cells that have to last a lifetime, such as the cells that make up the heart, the retina of the eye, and the nerve cells in the brain. Problems associated with this process include atherosclerosis, macular degeneration, and several neurodegenerative diseases, such as Alzheimer's disease.

Too many cells—Cells can get so old or damaged they can

no longer divide, but they also don't die and make room for others to divide—they kind of sit around consuming resources and don't contribute anything (many of us have friends and family members just like this, but that's another story). These senescent cells are inflammatory and are more vulnerable to the spread of cancer.

Too few cells—Some cells types die faster than they can be replaced. Over time, this can pose serious problems affecting the heart, the brain, and the immune system.

Genetic mutations—Several cancers are caused by this problem.

Mitochondrial mutations—Mitochondria are the energy-producing nuclear power plants that live inside our cells and have their own DNA. The process of converting food into energy spews out toxic waste called free radicals and bangs up mitochondrial DNA resulting in their ultimate demise.

Too many connections—Cells will develop abnormal bridges within and to each other causing tissues to lose elasticity. This causes arteries to stiffen (high blood pressure) and the lens of your eye to not play nice (it losses flexibility and that's why you eventually need reading glasses all over your house that you always lose).

Aging starts with a few cells here and there, then spreads to entire organ systems. This is manifested early on as age-associated annoyances like gray hair, age spots, and wrinkles. Later, , it can progress to degenerative conditions such as cardiovascular disease, diabetes, obesity, dementia, and cancer. This progression of a few cells losing their "maintenance contract" to full-blown organ system involvement takes time. This explains why most chronic diseases occur when we are older.

Several other processes are thought to contribute to why and how we age:

INFLAMMATION

Many experts claim that inflammation is the mother of all disease. Inflammation is supposed to be a good thing—it was designed to help you fight off germs and respond to injury. It was also designed to be a temporary response—to assist in the healing response. Once the threat is gone, inflammation ideally would be put to bed.

But for several reasons, inflammation sometimes gets stuck in the *on* position. Rather than healing, chronic inflammation causes cell damage and is debilitating. What causes chronic inflammation? Several things that are under your control such as obesity, smoking, eating crappy food, lack of exercise or activity, chronic stress, exposure to toxins (bug spray, gasoline fumes, household cleaning products, lack of sleep, nutritional deficiencies, and hormonal deficiencies).

CARMELIZATION

Well, not really, but sort of. We live in a world full of simple carbs (SUGAR), causing multiple blood sugar spikes throughout the day *every day*. This chronically elevated blood sugar drapes a syrupy coating over the biomolecules in our system. This causes these critical molecules to be sticky and thus, dysfunctional, negatively affecting almost every system in the body.

GENETIC COMMAND AND CONTROL PROBLEMS

Although it has been argued that it takes millions of years for genetic shifts and mutations to occur in a given species to affect what and who we are, we now know that lifestyle choices can flip the individual "switches" which control *access* to the genes in our DNA. So, although our DNA remains true to form, what individual genes get turned on (or off) and to what extent can be largely determined by your lifestyle. This is the field of epigenetics. Research has even shown that a bad lifestyle can have genetic implications that are passed down to your children in the womb!

LIMITED NUMBER OF CELL DIVISIONS

Telomeres act to maintain the integrity of chromosomes. They facilitate cell every day cell division and keep large DNA strands from sticking together end on end. In 1960, a famous scientist named Leonard Hayflick proposed that normal cells could only replicate or double fifty times. This is because the telomeres at the end of chromosomes shorten each time a cell divides. After a maximum of fifty divisions, the telomeres become too short to allow for cell division. Thus, according to Dr. Hayflick, the cells of our body have a finite lifespan, even in perfect conditions. This is known as the "Hayflick limit."

OXIDATIVE STRESS ("METABOLIC RUST")

An *oxygen free radical* is a "waste product" of normal metabolism, like the exhaust of an engine. It's the price our cells pay just to function. We have several natural "antioxidants" in our body that serve to keep our oxidation load finely balanced and tuned. Too much oxidation is called *oxidative stress*. Toxic buildup of these free radicals damages our DNA and disrupts our cellular "housekeeping." As we age, the accumulated effects of free radical damage take their toll. Several things cause oxidative stress including obesity, smoking, eating crappy food, and lack of exercise or activity.

AUTOIMMUNE SENESCENCE

With age, our body loses its ability to produce the necessary antibodies to fight disease—as well as its ability to distinguish *itself* from foreign invaders. The immune system becomes self-destructive and reacts against itself—the basis of several autoimmune diseases like rheumatoid arthritis, lupus, and thyroid disease (Hashimotos disease). Research has even suggested that high "bad" cholesterol is an autoimmune response to several factors that are influenced by lifestyle.

THE NEUROENDOCRINE THEORY

Hormones are secreted by glands under the direction of chemicals in the brain. Hormones orchestrate regulation and repair of important bodily functions. If your hormones are being produced at youthful levels, the cells of your body are encouraged to be active and stay young. The neuroendocrine theory states that a major cause of aging is malfunction of the brain's control over our glands, resulting in hormone deficiencies. In other words, the brain's command and control system over the glands is broken and nobody is stearing the ship. Thus, the body loses its ability to regulate and repair itself. This theory suggests that we age because our hormones decline; our hormones do not decline because we age.

We all know that some people take the aging hit earlier and faster than others. There can be a surprising difference between chronological age (your actual age) and biological age (how you look, feel, and function). How many times have you seen people who look ten years older than their age? We all know a few "Doogie Howsers" who seem to be gleefully sipping from the fountain of youth (and it's kind of irritating sometimes--in an envious sort of way). Discovering your biological age (more on that later) can serve as a wakeup call that motivates you to change your direction and put the brakes on aging *proactively.*

WHERE ARE YOU ON THE AGE CURVE?

Other than your appearance, there are some pretty fancy tests available to actually measure your biological age (although some people would rather not know!). Your biological age is a good thing to know because it gives you a snapshot of how well (or poorly) you are playing the aging game and if there is room for improvement to prevent the onset of the many chronic de-generative diseases that are in your 'biological horizon'.

Here's how it works:

An intensive physical examination combined with a battery of diagnostic tests measures how each of your organs are working. You can actually assess the "biological age" of your heart, lungs, skin, immune system, bones, and even your brain (including new and exciting ways to evaluate cognitive function and neuropsychological status—all pretty cool brain stuff).

Telomere test—This test measures the length of your telomeres. Telomeres are protective caps at the end of your chromosomes, kind of like the plastic tips at the end of shoelaces, that the cell machinery grabs onto when it's time to duplicate itself for growth and maintenance. They also keep your DNA for 'hooking up' end to end to form large non-sense strands (you would think that DNA would be smarter than that). Every time your cell divides, you lose a little piece of your telomeres. Eventually, telomeres get so short that the cell can no longer reproduce, and eventually it either dies or hangs around indefinitely contributing nothing while consuming resources. The faster and "dirtier" you burn your biological engine over the years due to a poor lifestyle and acquired illnesses, the shorter your telomeres will be . . . and the older you are biologically (long telomeres are a good thing).

HOW CAN YOU OUTSMART AGING?

Throughout this book, I will take you on a journey to discover several ways to slow—and in some cases, reverse—the effects of aging on your health and appearance. The potential lifespan of humans may possibly exceed 120 years. To achieve this, you must have a healthy mind, body, and spirit. The medical "know how" to achieve this has arrived. Small changes over time make a big difference. So let's get started.

". . . at the beginning a disease is more difficult to diagnose and easy to cure. But as time passes, not having been treated or recognized at the outset, it becomes easy to diagnose but difficult to cure."

—Niccoló Machiavelli, *The Prince*

CHAPTER 2

WHAT ARE HORMONES AND WHY SHOULD I CARE?

"Don't think of hormones as hot flashes, think of them as your inner child playing with matches!" —ANONYMOUS

Most physicians in the United States know surprisingly little about hormones and how they work. As physicians we receive a basic overview in medical school about which hormone each gland secretes, and we have a fundamental understanding of what these hormones do. The main focus of our "hormone education" is confined to learning the various awful disease states that occur when hormones run awry.

Endocrinologists, who specialize in hormone diseases, are masters at diagnosing and treating bad things that affect your endocrine glands and the hormones they secrete. Hormone optimization, however, wasn't included in their curriculum because nobody seemed to know too much about it or cared . . . endocrine disease is their focus . . . That's kind of surprising, isn't it?

Until recently, if your hormone levels fell within a non-specific "normal range," then you were considered "healthy."

However, we now know that "normal" hormone levels can be woefully inadequate to support your particular unique physiology. Although not in the "illness" range that most doctors use before they take action, even seemingly normal levels can significantly impact your quality of life and set you up for acquiring chronic disease in the future. What are healthy levels for an 18 year old Asian female may not be the same as for a 56 year old black male. *Not being sick does NOT mean you are healthy!!*

THE SIGNIFICANCE OF HORMONES

I'll never forget the story of an amazing woman I once knew. Sadly, she had lost her father suddenly, when he suffered cardiac arrest. She had such a difficult time seeing him alive one day and lifeless the next.

Later that year she was persuaded by her doctor to have a hysterectomy and removal of her ovaries due to some health issues that concerned him. She followed doctor's orders and had the surgery, but didn't feel good about going through with it.

As we discussed this procedure a month later, she related the loss of her "female organs" to the death of her father. She said that although she was alive, she felt dead inside. Her eyes didn't sparkle like they used to, and her smile was oftentimes a frown those days. She felt as if the life had been removed from her. Truth be told, the vital force of several important hormones had been quickly snatched from her. Her message to anyone who would listen was to recognize how much hormones really do impact our lives.

You may not realize this until yours quit cooperating.

HORMONES 101

The major endocrine glands include the following:

- pituitary
- thyroid
- parathyroid
- adrenal
- pancreas
- testicles
- ovaries

Hormones are part of a complex messenger system that is secreted into your bloodstream by your glands. They travel to all the cells of your body controlling many critical bodily functions. These functions include growth and development, repair, metabolism, reproduction, sexual function, mental function, and mood.

Hormones interact with each other in a complex, interdependent web. Suboptimal levels in one hormone can create havoc with other hormones simultaneously, creating a domino effect. These hormones are very powerful. Small changes in blood levels can cause big problems, both short- and long-term.

Our bodies are crafted like a finely tuned Swiss watch. All of the components must fit and function together perfectly to show the correct "time." A malfunction of any component, even a small one, can cause time to stop. The delicate balance of your hormones plays a big role in how your body performs, how well you feel, and your overall health.

Unfortunately, and for many different reasons, hormones become unbalanced as we age. Testosterone, estrogen, progesterone, growth hormone, and thyroid hormone levels can decrease, while insulin and cortisol hormones usually increase. These changes, though not defined as *disease* by the medical community, contribute significantly to the aging process resulting in the physical and mental changes we observe as people age. It also influences how we feel on a daily basis. As a matter of fact, we can point the finger at hormonal changes for heralding many of the chronic, age-related diseases common in our Western culture. These include cardiovascular disease, obesity, diabetes, osteoporosis, dementia, and even cancer.

We generally shrug our shoulders and tell ourselves that it's just all part of getting older. We blame bad genes, or bad luck, when our quality of life declines or chronic disease comes knocking.

Believe it or not, though, there is good news! Although hormones can fall, the cells in our bodies retain their ability to respond to hormones if they are replaced! This means that if we can replace these hormones to optimal levels, we can help put the brakes on the aging process. By replacing hormones we can help slow the onset of age-related diseases years before they appear—or even prevent them altogether. The trick to doing this is to use bioidentical hormone replacement therapy early to nudge these hormones back to where they need to be.

THE PROCESS OF HORMONE REPLACEMENT THERAPY

We are all similar physiologically, but each of us has a unique biochemistry. So how do physicians determine exactly where these hormone levels need to be? We have different ethnic backgrounds, family histories, body structure, psychological profiles, stress levels, and lifetime exposure to various environmental toxins. This makes our biochemistry as unique as our fingerprint.

All of these variables must be included in a physician's mental calculus when treating hormone imbalances. This means that a one-size-fits-all approach won't work. What works for one individual may not work for another.

Physicians managing hormone problems must have a very detailed picture of your family background, medical and surgical history, social and work environment, diet, fitness regimen, and a candid confession of your "bad habits." That's right, grab your diary . . . You have to spill the beans on habits you may not be too proud of! Detailed discussions on seemingly trivial symptoms and complaints are critical. Comprehensive laboratory evaluations that measure hormones and their metabolites complete the picture. This allows the physician to craft a program unique to your needs.

Typically, after a hormone program is prescribed, symptoms and hormone levels are closely followed, and the treatment plan is fine-tuned as needed. This requires a close working relationship with the physician and may take several months to accomplish. Symptoms usually abate relatively quickly. Alterations in dosing may also be necessary, depending on changes in lifestyle and health status.

SYNTHETIC HORMONES: NOT REALLY HORMONES AT ALL

A major flaw in many hormone replacement therapy programs prescribed today entails the use of synthetic hormones. Synthetic hormones are not really hormones at all . . . They are hormone-like substances, or imposters.

In order for big pharmaceutical companies to patent a drug, they must chemically alter the hormone molecule to make it unique. They can't patent a natural compound found in nature (Mother Nature already has dibs). The result is a molecule that is just a bit *off*—it doesn't quite fit the natural hormone receptors in the cell. This misfit can have terrible side effects. Several studies have shown that synthetic hormones have numerous adverse side effects that have been erroneously attributed to hormone replacement therapy using bioidentical hormones.

Bioidentical hormones are chemically the same as those naturally secreted by your glands. They fit into the specialized hormone receptors of your cells perfectly. The effects are identical to the effects of your natural hormones. Replacing hormones with the same thing that has surged throughout your body since birth is the only safe, effective way to manage deficiencies.

The benefits of bioidentical hormone replacement therapy are scientifically proven and irrefutable. Pay special attention to the word *irrefutable*. As part of a comprehensive age management program, we can help alleviate many the problems previously chalked up to "getting older."

Hormone replacement therapy may help you to:
- reclaim the energy and stamina you had in earlier years;
- improve your bodily functions, both physically and mentally, well beyond your current state; and
- avoid acquiring many of the chronic diseases that plague Western cultures (such as cardiovascular disease, stroke, cancer, osteoporosis, and dementia).

Quite simply, BHRT may help you achieve a more rewarding quality of life—to be your *absolute best*. The science is *irrefutable*; the technology is established. All you have to do is step up and raise your hand.

CHAPTER 3

MENOPAUSE, PERIMENOPAUSE AND OTHER FEMALE CONUNDRUMS

Women live most of their reproductive lives cycling monthly through the ebb and flow of estrogen and progesterone peaks and valleys. Many women teasingly call this "the curse." Any man who takes his eye off the ball, for even a moment, and minimalizes the relevance of this primal rhythm is playing with fire (or *hot flashes!*). He will be acutely reminded of the steep price to pay when his understanding of and lack of sensitivity to this fundamental cycle is forgotten or ignored.

However, the menstrual cycle is as natural as sunrise and rain. This well-choreographed dance of interdependent hormones is tightly regulated and designed with the engineering precision of a fine Swiss watch. As women age, this "watch" quits keeping time. Hormones stray from optimal levels and balance is lost. Even mild declines in one or two hormones can initiate to a system-wide "tilt" and upset this delicate balance, with far- ranging consequences in quality of life. The long-term health consequences can be quite significant.

There are support forums all over the Internet where women experiencing the changes and effects of menopause share their stories. One such story was written by a woman who was really struggling physically and emotionally because of her hormonal imbalances. Her story relates the significant impact hormones can have on your life—and even your marriage:

> *Hi All, I have written a few times on this board, and am waiting for my OB/Gyn to call me back. I am taking Prozac for Depression/Anxiety, and I have severe PMS. I had my blood work done, and the OB nurse said my thyroid was normal, but my estradiol level was low. It was only 20? Last year it was in the 90s!*
>
> *I have absolutely NO SEX drive whatsoever! Sex hurts and I could care less, and this is NOT FAIR to my husband at all. I have been married twenty-two years this coming December, and I know he is frustrated about this. I am worried. I am tired, still depressed and no sex drive—What can I do, or buy? Is there a medication for women that can help? I am 46 and was told I am not in menopause, but let me tell you, I think I am pre-menopausal. Last month's period had all the same PMS systems but was very light flow and black/brown in color.*
>
> *I am worried all the way around and don't know what to do. I am running out of options. I don't want to lose the love of my life and want to feel better. Please anyone. I need some help, advice, etc. This is not fair to him, and I need a better quality of life.*

In her mid-30s, a woman's hormones begin to decline. The timing and extent of this fall depends on several things:
- heredity
- lifestyle

- diet
- stress history
- other illnesses
- level of physical activity
- accumulated effects of our toxic environment

Eventually, a woman will begin to notice symptoms related to these hormonal changes. The fancy medical name for this phenomenon is called perimenopause. This can start as early as age 35 and can last for up to fifteen years. In time, the hormonal decline will result in cessation of a menstrual period. This is called menopause and is confirmed medically when there have been no periods for twelve consecutive months and no other biological or physiological cause can be identified. The timing of this event varies from woman to woman, but menopause usually occurs in the early 50s.

Both men and women are living longer these days. The average age of death for women in 1900 was 46 years of age. Now it is not uncommon for women to live to age 78 and beyond. This means that many women will live over forty years in a hormonally deficient state if untreated. That's forty years . . . half of their adult life! That's a long time to suffer from the symptoms of low hormone levels.

To make matters worse, we now know that these hormones are critical in helping to protect women from acquiring several chronic diseases such as breast cancer, uterine cancer, heart disease, Alzheimer's disease, autoimmune disease, diabetes, and weight gain. The good news is that this process can now be managed medically using bioidentical hormone replacement therapy. These important hormones can be measured in the blood, saliva, or urine and replaced in a balanced fashion by physician experts trained in this field.

The operative phrase here is "physician experts trained in

this field." This is a relatively new knowledge base that is not taught in medical school or in specialty training. Being a traditionally trained physician myself, I am aware that many of my physician peers simply don't have the background necessary to address these problems effectively and safely. We were all trained as disease doctors, not wellness doctors.

Traditionally, doctors have been trained to identify and treat disease—not to address and recognize subtle hormonal issues to optimize health (and insurance coverage for this "luxury" is non-existent—for now). This includes many endocrinologists, OB/Gyn physicians, internists, and family practice doctors. Much of their training, and most of their medical literature, is either directly or indirectly influenced by large pharmaceutical corporations. The traditional tools available to most physicians are limited to either surgery or synthetic pharmaceuticals.

When the need for hormone replacement IS recognized, people are then categorized and labeled with a disease, and in an algorithmic "pill for every ill" mindset, prescribed a synthetic hormone product. The doctor may even go on to reassure the patient that this is just what happens when you get older, prescribing medications for sleep, anxiety, and depression or recommending intrusive surgery to remove the "offending organs" (uterus and ovaries). This way, a woman can just be done with the whole mess once and for all.

In today's time-crunched, volume-driven medical business environment, many physicians just don't have the time, inclination, or expertise to handle these situations in a personalized way. Doctors must tease out many delicate and subtle intricacies to address the sometimes obscure nature of hormonal imbalances—skills many practitioners lack. There is a better way!

A balanced program of bioidentical hormone replacement therapy, healthy nutrition, stress management, and regular exercise can yield amazing results. The emerging fields of integrative medicine and age management have revolutionized our ability to revive and maintain wellness, permitting us to age better. Not only can we help make postmenopausal years more enjoyable, but hopefully, we can help protect you from the chronic health conundrums that befall many in our society. Before we get started, let's talk a little bit about the normal menstrual cycle (*and don't worry: I'll try not to get too technical!*).

THE MENSTRUAL CYCLE-MORE THAN YOU EVER WANTED TO KNOW

Before we delve into what happens to a woman's reproductive system as she ages, let's briefly review the normal nuts and bolts of the menstrual cycle. This cycle is designed to prepare the lining of the uterus to receive and nurture a fertilized egg . . . to make more of us!

The sequence of events leading to this event is controlled by a small part of the brain called the pituitary gland. This little gland secretes chemicals into the blood which travel to the ovaries, "commanding" them to increase production of the hormone estrogen Increased production of estrogen by the ovaries causes the uterine lining to thicken, creating a nice cozy bed in anticipation of receiving a fertilized egg.

The little pituitary gland also stimulates the ovaries to produce a suitable, mature, egg that will eventually pop out of the ovary into the fallopian tube (the highway to the uterus). This process is called ovulation and takes place at around the 14th day of the cycle. The mature egg then starts its journey down the fallopian tube, waiting for a "date" with an appropriate sperm suitor.

The egg leaves behind its previous home in the ovary, a little sack now renamed the corpus luteum, which begins to make progesterone. This further enhances the uterus' cozy lining in anticipation of pregnancy (the ultimate optimist).

I mean, this really *is* a team effort! If, after approximately seventy-two hours, a fertilized egg does not arrive on the scene, that little ovarian sack stops producing progesterone, and the lining of the uterus simply sloughs away in what most women know as their "period." This process repeats itself over and over every month throughout a female's reproductive years.

CHANGES IN THE MENSTRUAL CYCLE AS WOMEN AGE

As a woman enters her mid-30s, both her brain and her ovaries begin to lose their effectiveness in manufacturing the "baby-making" substances necessary to orchestrate this monthly cycle. When this occurs, menstrual irregularities begin to manifest, and several new symptoms arise that begin to affect quality of life.

These symptoms can be quite subtle, confusing and frequently atypical, leading to a delayed or improper diagnosis and ineffective treatment. Many women are told that they are stressed, depressed, anxious, or even crazy and are provided a colorful assortment of psychotropic drugs to get them through their day. This is how many women are ushered into the phenomenon that we know as perimenopause.

PERIMENOPAUSE-AGING KNOCKING AT YOUR DOOR

The first hormone that typically declines as women age is progesterone. This occurs in the late 30s to early 40s. One of the many important jobs of progesterone is to balance the effects of estrogen on the body—it keeps estrogen in check! You can think of estrogen and progesterone as "yin and yang" hormones having many opposite effects.

When progesterone drops, yin has deserted yang, and estrogen is now unopposed, leading to a power play situation called estrogen dominance . . . too much estrogen relative to progesterone. This "estrogen dominance" is responsible for most of the nasty symptoms experienced by women in perimenopause. The symptoms of perimenopause can precede menopause by five to ten years (oh my!).

To add insult to injury, negative lifestyle choices can exacerbate estrogen dominance. Fat cells produce estrogen, and too many fat cells (obesity) is a well-known cause of estrogen dominance. Synthetic estrogens (xeno-estrogens) are everywhere in our environment and can be found in plastics, food, cosmetics, and insecticides.

As we approach menopause, estrogen production eventually becomes erratic. The ovaries start to sputter. Testosterone falls. Our three most important sex hormones (estrogen, progesterone, and testosterone) begin to falter. This ushers in a whole host of unpleasant symptoms, making daily life quite uncomfortable. Most importantly, women now become vulnerable to several preventable age-related chronic diseases if this hormonal imbalance is not dealt with.

MENOPAUSE—BLESSING OR CURSE?

You have "officially" entered menopause when you have gone one year without a menstrual period. Early in menopause, you may still be estrogen dominant, but eventually, estrogen levels will fade and estrogen, progesterone, and testosterone may all be significantly deficient. Now you are deficient in all of the sex hormones. This is the time when women need comprehensive support.

WHAT DOES IT FEEL LIKE TO HAVE LOW ESTROGEN AND PROGESTERONE?

How many women have suffered from PMS? Remember how bad you felt just before your period? Remember how it affected your mood? Would it surprise you to know that PMS results from a relative deficiency of progesterone? Would it really irritate you to know that a little added progesterone, just a dab of cream or pill once a day, could have rescued you from years of aggravation?

The symptoms of early perimenopause are similar to the symptoms one experiences with PMS. After all, the reasons for both are the same—estrogen dominance. There are several classical symptoms of perimenopause, but there are also many vague and obscure symptoms that can be confusing. Without a high index of suspicion, symptoms of perimenopause can be missed or misinterpreted and appropriate treatment delayed.

Everyone is familiar with the obvious symptoms of perimenopause: irritability, hot flashes, irregular periods, and weight gain. In fact, over 75 percent of all perimenopausal and menopausal women suffer from hot flashes. Symptoms can, however, be obscure and tricky. Consider this list of common, yet surprisingly unknown, symptoms of perimenopause that I see in my office every day:

- depression, anxiety
- short-term memory loss
- sleep disturbances, fatigue
- migraines
- breast pain, breast cysts
- weight gain, fluid retention, and food cravings
- joint pain
- breakthrough bleeding, heavy menstrual bleeding
- bloating

• uterine fibroids, ovarian cysts

These are not symptoms typically associated with perimenopause, but they are important and can have a huge impact on quality of life. What is really BIG is that these symptoms can PRECEDE menopause by ten years! More bad news . . . many traditional doctors will flip you a Xanax or anti-depressant to get you through your hormone-deprived day! Although those around you may appreciate this, it is not a good solution.

As you progress along perimenopausal trail toward menopause, estrogen starts to fade, and you begin to see the effects of low estrogen, progesterone, and testosterone as well: the trifecta of hormonal abandonment. The female urinary tract and vagina may thin out, leading to urinary incontinence, bladder infections, and vaginal dryness. Your skin will begin to thin and become dry, blotchy, wrinkled, and easily damaged. Libido tends to go on permanent holiday. Energy levels decline, and morning sluggishness or 3 p.m. energy dips can be a real problem. Brain fog sets in and mental acuity can get a little sloppy (where did I leave my keys?). Depression or anxiety can become more pronounced, exacerbated by fatigue.

WHY "TREAT" PERIMENOPAUSE AND MENOPAUSE?

Many people feel that the symptoms of menopause and perimenopause, although unpleasant, are just part of getting older. Are there any compelling reasons why we need to proactively address the "change of life?"

Absolutely! Mountains of research confirm that bioidentical hormone replacement therapy can play a big role in preventing several chronic age-related diseases and are instrumental in maintaining health and vitality. And, most importantly, it can make a woman feel like a million dollars!

ESTROGEN

Why should we use estrogen? Estrogen has proven beneficial in collagen production for thicker skin, vagina and bladder tissue elasticity, and heart valve health. Estrogen is important in the prevention of heart disease and stroke. It is a powerful antioxidant, helping combat free radicals and their effects in the aging process. Estrogen stimulates skeletal growth and maintains healthy bones; it has also been shown to increase HDL cholesterol. Estrogen supports brain function, maximizes critical thinking, and stabilizes mood. Estrogen supplementation increases insulin sensitivity, helping to prevent adult onset diabetes. Enough said!

Take this simple quiz to see if you may be suffering from the effects of low estrogen:
www.IntegrativeMedicineDallas/lowestrogen_quiz.com

PROGESTERONE

As already noted, progesterone balances estrogen. Since progesterone is the first sex hormone to decline as we age, it should be the first one we replace to avoid estrogen dominance. By the age of 40, the average American female has lost 80 percent of her progesterone. Remember, estrogen dominance can result in several disruptive symptoms and also makes women susceptible to abnormal growths such as cancer, fibroids, and cysts.

There are progesterone receptors in every tissue in the body, not just the uterus. Progesterone plays a very important role in all tissues. Not having a uterus does not mean you can pass on progesterone therapy. Progesterone helps estrogen build and maintain bones. Progesterone also protects the heart, blood vessels, and nerves. It has been referred to as the "feel-good hormone" and can have a profound effect on the brain, acting as a calming agent, relieving anxiety and moodiness, and facilitating restful sleep. It is also been shown to help obviate menopausal depression.

Interestingly, women under constant stress can be progesterone deficient without being perimenopausal. Constant stress creates chronically elevated levels of the stress hormone cortisol. Since cortisol and progesterone are made from the same building blocks, prolonged high cortisol production from stress steals more than its fair share of those blocks, resulting in progesterone getting the short end of the stick. This can result in many of the same symptoms as a woman undergoing early menopause due to estrogen dominance (*See how tricky this stuff is?*).

Try this quiz to see if you are progesterone deficient:
www.IntegrativeMedicineDallas/lowprogesterone_quiz.com

TESTOSTERONE

Testosterone is not just for men. Women need it too, just not as much. Around 30 percent of a woman's testosterone is produced in the ovary along with estrogen and progesterone. The remaining 70 percent is derived from the adrenal gland (which sits on top of the kidneys). Testosterone levels peak in a woman in her 20s and then decrease with each passing year. At menopause, a woman's testosterone is at an all-time low.

This testosterone drop and its related symptoms are magnified by the effects of estrogen and progesterone deficiency. Testosterone has the glorious effect of sparking a healthy libido, which is usually missing in action in an aging female. A great libido is a nice little side effect, but testosterone does several other important things for us as well. Testosterone helps revitalize skin texture. Testosterone has a big effect on muscle mass, increasing strength and consumption of calories, decreasing the accumulation of body fat. It works with estrogen to prevent osteoporosis. Low testosterone can cause poor memory, foggy thinking, and contribute toward low libido, depression, heart disease, and dementia! Replacing it is a very good thing, indeed.

BIOIDENTICAL HORMONE REPLACEMENT—THE BASICS

Treatment of female hormone deficiencies begins with a comprehensive medical history, comprehensive physical exam and a detailed laboratory evaluation. As I have previously stated, hormone systems are interdependent, and deficiencies or excesses in one system can affect other systems in profound ways—so we need to look at everything.

For example, a malfunctioning thyroid gland or high cortisol levels from chronic stress can affect estrogen and testosterone levels. Fixing one problem without addressing the others will fail—and it's not uncommon to find multiple hormonal system imbalances at the same time. That is why drawing a full laboratory panel, including an analysis of all hormones, is essential before any effort is made to diagnose and treat problems.

The most important part of the evaluation is the initial consultation. A careful history and physical examination, along with thoughtful and intimate questioning to tease out any subtle symptoms, tells the story and leads to a diagnosis. The consultation is a warm, fuzzy time when the subjective "intangibles" are laid out for scrutiny and open, frank discussion. Most of the time, a laboratory evaluation serves only to confirm our diagnosis and acts as a yardstick to dose the medication and manage the specifics.

Bioidentical hormone replacement therapy (BHRT) uses hormones whose molecular structure is identical to that of humans. Bioidentical hormones fit human physiology perfectly—like a lock and key. Synthetic estrogens and progesterone, used by many physicians who don't know better, are dangerous drugs, as several studies have clearly demonstrated. They need to be avoided at all costs!

We need to get mainstream physicians up to speed and out from under the biased influence of pharmaceutical manufacturers, myth, dogma, and un-enlightened tradition. Today's rapidly changing healthcare landscape may make the "schooling" of our healthcare provider brothers and sisters imperative as social and financial pressures dictate the shift from treatment of disease to promotion of health.

BHRT—HOW WE DO IT

For estrogen replacement, we recommend creams. Creams are demonstrably the most consistent delivery method, as well as the safest. Estrogen pills, while convenient, result in metabolic changes that can be harmful. Oral estrogen passes immediately through the liver, with several possible adverse effects. These include increased triglycerides, insulin resistance, elevated blood pressure, gallbladder disease, and increased risk of cancer from carcinogenic by-products.

Oral estrogen can also result in the production of clotting factors that increase the chance of developing blood clots in the legs, leading to a potentially fatal pulmonary embolus. We see no logical reason why anyone would ever possibly consider estrogen pills.

None of these negative effects have arisen with creams. Creams are applied to the skin overlying fatty portions of the thighs or belly, where they dissolve into the underlying fat and are slowly released to the body steadily throughout the day. Estrogen can also be applied vaginally if desired. The downside of creams is that absorption can be erratic (although this is rare). It is also possible to transfer estrogen to husbands, children, or pets if you're not careful. All of that being said, estrogen creams are, for most women, the way to go.

Some clinics advocate estrogen pellets. Pellets sure are convenient (in theory), but in my expert opinion, the risks outweigh the benefits. Pellets have a documented sterility problem depending on where they're manufactured. Pellet placement is a surgical procedure that is not always performed by someone who is surgically skilled. Additionally, the surgical procedure must be repeated every three to five months for an indefinite time period (twenty years–how long to you want to feel good?). That's a lot of surgery, with many chances for bruising, scarring, and infection. Finally, placing pellets is relatively inflexible with regard to dosing. If a chosen dose of estrogen is too strong, you're kind of stuck with it . . . literally!

Progesterone can be prescribed as a cream or a pill. The nice thing about progesterone cream is that it can be combined with the estrogen cream, which makes things easier. Progesterone pills are great and don't have the nasty liver side effects seen with estrogen pills. Plus, when taken at night, progesterone pills serve as a convenient sleep aid. We think pills are the way to go for most women.

Testosterone replacement for women is best achieved using daily creams. On rare occasion, creams just don't cut it, and other methods can be used (such as low-dose injections or vaginal suppositories). Almost all women do great with testosterone creams.

THE FOLLOW-UP

After hormone therapy begins, we see our patients in three months to evaluate the effectiveness of their treatment and to get follow-up labs. At that time, any necessary dose adjustments are made. Once we discover the right mix and dose, we do check-ups every six months. It's important to remember that your body is in a continual state of change, and your physiological needs change from time to time. This can be due to changes in season, stress levels, weight, the addition of other medications, illnesses, new exercise program, a new boyfriend, a new house, or a new job. Nearly anything can have an impact on hormone levels.

LONG-TERM PLAN

It's not uncommon for patients to ask me, "Hey Doc, how long do I have to be on this stuff?" The answer is simple: how long do you want to feel great and stay healthy? Hormone therapy is intended to replace youthful levels of hormones to keep us rocking and rolling at our best *indefinitely*. I have patients in their 80s who are pushing forward with no end in sight!

BIOCHEMICAL HORMONES: MYTHS AND FACTS

Some women may be reluctant to embrace bioidentical hormone therapy. This concern is based on an ill-conceived study called the "Women's Health Initiative," a fifteen-year study conducted by the US National Institutes of Health. This study measured several things. A subset of the study evaluated the effects of hormone replacement therapy on postmenopausal women and how it affected their health. The study was halted prematurely, in 2002, with the conclusion that the associated health risk of combined hormone therapy was dangerous and should be abandoned!

These results were highly publicized. Many doctors and the lay press warned women against the dangers of hormone replacement therapy. Since the release of these findings, the study has been scrutinized and re-evaluated time and time again. Several flaws in its design, which led to unsound conclusions, have been highlighted in journal after journal. The most blatant flaw was that the project studied only postmenopausal women using only synthetic hormones. Of course, a study of postmenopausal women using artificial hormone-like drugs tells us nothing about the value bioidentical hormones in both perimenopausal and postmenopausal women.

Comparing synthetic hormones to bioidentical hormones is like comparing the REAL Elvis Presley to the Las Vegas Elvis that you see in every Vegas casino. Each cell in the body has a specific, unique receptor for every hormone. This is true for estrogen and progesterone. They need the real thing.

These receptors have to be "unlocked" with the perfect key in order for a natural, desired effect to be achieved. That perfect key is Mother Nature's own biologically perfect estrogen and progesterone. Premarin, Provera, and other hormonal "imposters" manufactured by pharmaceutical companies just don't fit these receptors. In fact, the fit is usually shaky at best. These "hormone-like" substances are foreign invaders in our system and provoke a whole shopping list of adverse side effects. These adverse side effects are what were observed in the infamous "Women's Health Initiative," and the literature of the last five years is replete with new studies unequivocally demonstrating the safety, efficacy, and necessity of BHRT.

Despite the plethora of science supporting the many benefits of BHRT, many traditional doctors still caution their patients on the dangers of their use. Consider this common-sense challenge:

> *A 22-year-old female's body is surging with sky-high levels of estrogen, progesterone, and testosterone. Why don't these "dangerous" natural chemicals ravage these*

*young women? Why are high levels of estrogen, proges-
terone, and testosterone good and healthy for 22-year-old
women and poison for 50-year-old women? Why don't
we see breast cancer and increased heart disease in 22
year olds if hormones are indeed as toxic as indicated
by the "Women's Health Initiative" study? Why is it that
these problems become more prevalent in our female population only after these precious hormone levels plunge
(which typically occurs between the ages 50 and 60)?*

Replacing like with like, BHRT restores a more youthful biology, warding off premature aging and chronic disease. Common sense and contemporary research confirm that hormone
replacement therapy is a MUST if women desire to remain
healthy, vigorous, and robust.

CHAPTER 4

ANDROPAUSE: EVEN ROME FELL

A frustrated woman once asked her male friend why men act like jerks. His reply was, "It's a testosterone thing. Much similar to your PMS thing, we men suffer from testosterone poisoning. Why do you think the average life span of a male is typically ten years shorter (and it's not just from all the nagging we have to endure)? Hormone modifies behavior. We're just misunderstood." (http://www.jokebuddha.com)

WHEN A MAN'S HORMONES LEAVE THE BUILDING

Hormone decline is not just for women. Unfortunately, most men start to lose their hormones as well. Although testosterone is the big one that causes the most concern and receives the most attention, other hormones can also take a dive as men age.

Thyroid hormone, cortisone, and human growth hormone (HGH) declines can play a big part in your overall health and how you feel. Estrogen is another hormone that can cause problems for men. (And I will talk more about that later.) Package all these hormone imbalances into one big ball, and what you now have is something called andropause.

Many of the symptoms and health consequences of andropause are similar to those seen in women undergoing menopause. Most men will begin to feel the subtle changes of andropause in their early to mid-40s. Unlike women, these changes are often subtle and sneak up on men as they approach their 50s. Men begin to notice that they just don't have the energy they used to. Their sex drive takes a vacation. Their endurance while engaging in competitive sports is diminished. Their short-term memory starts to falter, and their mental sharpness gets a little fuzzy.

There are many symptoms that *scream* andropause. Review the following list and see if any of these apply to you:

- changes in hair growth patterns (loss of hair in some areas, or new hair appearing in places that you're not too happy about (like your ears);
- decreased or total lack of interest in sex;
- inability to obtain or maintain an erection;
- breast enlargement (commonly called "man boobs" but properly termed gynecomastia);
- weight gain and loss of muscle mass;
- inability to fall asleep or stay asleep;
- mood changes such as irritability or depression;
- decreased energy or outright fatigue;
- fuzzy thinking and impairment of intellectual performance;
- short-term memory loss; and
- loss of motivation and initiative.

TREATING WITH TESTOSTERONE—EVERYBODY DESERVES A SECOND CHANCE

With testosterone therapy, one's attitude improves. There is an increase in self-esteem and self-confidence, as well as increased energy. Most men will feel more vigorous, experience improved energy levels, mood, concentration, cognition, libido, sexual performance, and an overall sense of well-being. These effects are usually noted within three to six weeks.

Other potential medical benefits include lowering LDL cholesterol, decreased risk of cardiovascular disease, improved insulin sensitivity (which helps prevent diabetes), maintenance or improvement in bone density, improved body composition, and increased muscle mass and muscle strength, and improvement in visual-spatial skills and mentation.

Andropause is not just about hormones. Several issues, including how and what you eat, your activity level, your stress history, and the environmental toxins you accumulate in your body over the years are also players. We will address these issues separately in other chapters. For now, let's discuss testosterone deficiency.

Most men are unaware that their testosterone levels may drop as they enter their 40s and 50s. They just assume that the reason they feel the way they do is because they aren't spring chickens anymore. Most men will start to show a decline in their testosterone levels around age 25, and this continues gradually throughout life.

THE IMPORTANCE OF TESTOSTERONE

Having adequate testosterone levels in a man is huge. Testosterone plays a pivotal role in a man's health and well-being. Testosterone is critically important for maintaining muscle mass. Adequate levels also protect the heart and are instrumental in preventing cardiovascular disease. Testosterone is also necessary for brain health and can be a critical cofactor in helping to prevent the onset of dementia and Alzheimer's disease. Healthy testosterone levels play an important role in quashing the onset of type II diabetes—a condition that is epidemic in American

Westernized culture. Deficiencies in testosterone can negatively affect almost every system in your body. This deficiency is a setup for the development of several chronic diseases that we would all rather avoid.

PHYSIOLOGY: TESTOSTERONE 101

As most men know, testosterone is made primarily in the testicles. What many men may not know is that testosterone production is driven by the brain. Little messengers secreted from a gland called the pituitary travel through the bloodstream to the testicles instructing them to make testosterone and sperm. When testosterone levels get too low, the brain will send more of these little messengers to tell the testicles to get to work.

Likewise, when testosterone gets too high, the pituitary messengers back off in an effort to bring testosterone levels back to normal. This becomes important with testosterone therapy. Why? When you add testosterone externally, the brain will sense this and feel like there is plenty of that wonderful testosterone stuff around and tells the testicles to take a vacation.

Another interesting little tidbit about testosterone is the manner in which it moves around the body. After testosterone is secreted by the testicles, most of it is attached to little carrier cars (called SHBG and albumin) which escort the testosterone where it needs to go. Once testosterone arrives at its destination, it detaches from the carriers and becomes "free testosterone." It's *free* testosterone that actually enters the cells and does the heavy lifting.

Theoretically, a man can have a normal *total* testosterone level, yet a high percentage of it is bound to these carriers, resulting in a low *free* testosterone. Several conditions can prevent testosterone from dissociating from its carriers, thus prevent entry into the cell where the work is done. These conditions have to be recognized and addressed for testosterone treatment to be effective.

As we've already mentioned, testosterone levels naturally start to decline in your mid to late-20s, and by the time you reach your 40s and 50s, they can be quite low. Testosterone deficiency has many causes. One easy way for physicians to determine if it's the testicles or the brain to blame for low testosterone is to measure the blood levels of the pituitary messengers (FSH and LH) that actually "talk" to the testicles. Low FSH, LH, and testosterone point to the brain, not the testicles, as the problem. In this case, the testicles are working fine and dandy but there is not enough FSH or LH around to cheer them on. A history of head trauma or chronic stress can derail the brain's secretion of FSH and LH, resulting in low testosterone secretion. That means all we have to do to fix it is to nudge the testicles to wake up and join the party.

Similarly, when testosterone treatment is given externally in the form of a cream, pellets, or injections, the pituitary senses that all is well in the testosterone universe and secretion of LH and FSH decreases. This tells the testicles to take a siesta and relax. Alternatively, if the testicles just aren't stepping up to the plate, the LH and FSH messengers levels will be high, which is the brain's way of screaming at them, "Hey dude, I need more testosterone!" In these cases, we can replace the testosterone hormone directly.

TESTOSTERONE DOES NOT ALWAYS STAY AS TESTOSTERONE!

CONVERSION TO DHT

When testosterone is secreted by the testicles or given therapeutically, some of it is converted into a compound with the long fancy name dihydrotestosterone, or DHT for short. DHT is an important chemical and is responsible for all things male. Male pattern hair growth (and unfortunately, *hair loss*), muscle mass, and genitalia development are all driven by DHT. DHT levels are relatively low in young men and tend to increase with age.

Sometimes DHT levels can creep up too high, resulting in unwanted side effects such as excessive hair loss, aggressive behavior, acne, and perhaps prostate enlargement, making urination difficult. Some people make more of this stuff than others. Monitoring DHT levels is very important in any hormone program designed to optimize testosterone levels.

DHT can be blocked using saw palmetto, pumpkin seeds or by using the drug finasteride. These remedies act to block the enzyme responsible for turning testosterone into DHT. Finasteride unfortunately has several side effects that are undesirable . . . like impotence and cognitive impairment. I tend not to use it (or use in very infrequently) since the potential problems outweigh the benefits.

CONVERSION TO ESTROGEN

Testosterone can also be converted by the body, through various chemical side reactions, into estrogen. Estrogen serves many important functions in males. As men age, more and more testosterone is diverted to estrogen. In fact, the average 60-year-old male has higher blood estrogen levels than the average 60-year-old female!

This increased estrogen can be responsible for the accumulation of excess body fat and the development of "man boobs" (gynecomastia). Several research papers have also implicated elevated estrogen levels as being responsible for prostate enlargement and an increased risk of prostate cancer. Elevated estrogen levels can also have detrimental effects on cardiovascular health.

Whether occurring naturally or as a result of hormone therapy, estrogen levels in the aging male need to be monitored, and if elevated, dealt with. Several natural and pharmacologic agents are available to keep estrogen values in the healthy range.

DIAGNOSING LOW TESTOSTERONE

The diagnosis of testosterone deficiency is based primarily on symptoms and then confirmed by laboratory evaluation. The trick is to figure out why testosterone is low. Is it due to the testicles underperforming? Is there a history of head trauma or chronic stress that throttled down the brain's secretion of testicle-stimulating LH and FSH? Is stress, with it's over the top production of cortisol, hogging all the chemical building blocks to make even more cortisol and leaving none for testosterone production? (More on this later . . . but this is why chronic stress can hit a man where he lives!!) Is testosterone disappearing because it is being turned into other things as it sloshes around the body (like DHT or estrogen)?

We use sequential lab tests to monitor testosterone treatment to ensure that testosterone is maintained at healthy levels—and that it is not being sidetracked into making DHT or estrogen. We also want to know that the bound testosterone can break away from its carrier protein (*"gets off the bus"*) as *free* testosterone once it reaches the cells. Finally, we monitor PSA to determine any possible adverse effects testosterone may be having on the prostate (although current research indicates that healthy levels of testosterone are actually protective against prostate cancer and prostate disease).

Note: *There are no studies that testosterone administration causes prostate cancer or an enlarged prostate. Testosterone levels are very high in young male adults. Why don't* *we see prostate cancer in young male adults if testosterone is toxic? Most traditional doctors have been trained to believe that testosterone increases the risk of prostate cancer. There is no data to support this.*

This should illustrate to even the most casual reader that the treatment of testosterone deficiency isn't a simple matter of adding a little testosterone to your system. It's important to figure out *why* the testosterone is low in the first place in order to treat it effectively. Once treatment starts, it's critical to find out where all this stuff is going and how the body is interacting with it in order to optimize its effects on your health and well-being while keeping you out of trouble.

At the very least, the following lab tests are the bare minimum required to assess and treat testosterone deficiency:

- complete blood count
- complete metabolic panel
- thyroid function studies
- total and free testosterone
- estrogen (estradiol)
- DHT (dihydrotestosterone)
- carrier proteins (SHBG and albumin)
- PSA

Ideally, a 24-hour saliva test to measure the levels of the stress hormone cortisol should also be obtained. One of the major causes of low testosterone is prolonged chronic stress, which elevates cortisol levels. This affects the brain's control over the testicles and steals the important building blocks required to make testosterone in the first place. The bottom line is: stress trashes your testosterone levels.

I have personal experience with this. At age 50, I decided to fulfill my desire to get an MBA. I picked one of the best schools in the country and away I went, still maintaining a medical practice! I was competing with 28-year-old geniuses. Consuming the information the professors demanded we learn was like drinking water from a fire hose. My stress was off the charts for two years. My testosterone eventually plummeted to one of the lowest levels I have ever seen—and I sure felt it! My energy and focus where off. My libido was zero (funny thing about libido—when it's low you don't care that it's low. When you don't have a sweet tooth—you don't miss it!)

As mentioned in an earlier chapter, the "normal" lab values for testosterone (and all hormones) may not be *optimal* for you. These normal ranges are derived from a very diverse population of thousands of people without consideration of age, body type, concurrent illnesses, or ethnic or cultural background. The ideal values we are looking for in diagnosis and treatment are generally those seen in a 30-year-old male in good health.

TESTOSTERONE REPLACEMENT THERAPY

Testosterone replacement can be accomplished in many different ways. You can use gels and creams, injections, discs placed under your tongue (sublingual), or pellets inserted into your fat. All of these methods have pros and cons.

GELS AND CREAMS

Gels and creams use testosterone initially extracted from soy or yams which is then processed to yield bioidentical human testosterone. They are easy to apply, provide stable blood levels throughout the day, quickly attain good serum levels, and closely mimic the body's natural testosterone secretion.

Gels are alcohol-based and limited in the amount of testosterone that can be transferred through the skin. On the other hand, creams are specifically designed to penetrate readily into the skin and can carry higher levels of testosterone to the body:

they are generally more efficient as a trans-dermal testosterone delivery method. It's important to avoid applying these products to hair-bearing areas since hair follicles can contain high levels of enzymes that convert testosterone to the undesirable DHT.

There is also a potential risk of accidental transfer to loved ones and pets, requiring you to be strategic about where you apply these agents. Finally, a small percentage of people have skin characteristics which make effective absorption of the medication difficult, though this is unusual. That being said, I feel that the creams are the easiest and most consistent method for testosterone supplementation. I personally prefer creams and use them in over 90 percent of my patients.

INJECTIONS (NOT AS BAD AS IT SOUNDS)

Traditionally, testosterone injections were given every two or three weeks. This created the problem of an initial surge of testosterone to super-high levels followed by dwindling levels in the days just prior to the next injection. So, part of the time testosterone is too high—part of the time it's too low. Testosterone dosing follows an efficiency curve. Ideally, we're trying to hit 'the sweet spot' with treatment. More is not better, and super-physiologic levels of testosterone can cause adverse health effects.

Most practitioners who use injections now give them on a weekly basis. This presents the same problem, although to a lesser degree. Some physicians (including me) are now prescribing smaller doses just under the skin twice a week. This method is very attractive, and I am beginning to use it in more of my patients. It's an effective way to minimize the initial surge followed by the lull in testosterone levels typically seen with weekly injections.

Injected testosterone converts more readily to estrogen, which as we have seen, has negative side effects. The advantage of testosterone injections is that of convenience, with essentially no risk of accidental transfer and full penetration into the bloodstream.

PELLETS

Another very popular testosterone delivery method utilizes several pellets surgically placed under the skin every three to four months. These pellets dissolve slowly and deliver a steady quantity of testosterone to the system.

Although popular and convenient, I personally have several problems with this approach. Like all surgical procedures, this is technique dependent and carries with it the risk of any surgical procedure including infection, bleeding or bruising, post-procedure pain, and scarring. Using surgery to administer hormone therapy seems a bit excessive to me (and I'm a surgeon). Testosterone requirements are also dynamic and may change with varying levels of stress, exercise, health status, and nutrition.

Pellet therapy does not allow for dynamic flexibility in short-term dosing on the part of the practitioner. If, for any reason, the implanted dose of testosterone pellets is too high, the only alternative available to adjust that dose is to remove the pellets! If the dose is too low—do you go back and insert a couple of more pellets? Also, just like weekly injections, the dose response in the blood is a big curve. The dose doesn't just turn off one day—it dwindles over the last couple of weeks to sub therapeutic levels. This means that there is a period of time when testosterone levels drop below what may be needed. Finally, it's not unusual for a patient to be on testosterone replacement therapy for years or even decades. The specter of undergoing a surgical procedure every three or four months for twenty years really makes no sense to me when easier, better methods exist.

HCG

HCG is short for human chorionic gonadotropin. This molecule closely resembles LH, the messenger from the brain to the testicles that we discussed earlier. Remember that LH is secreted by the pituitary in the brain to tell the testicles to wake up and crank out more testosterone. Also remember that when testosterone is given in therapy, the brain thinks all is well and shuts down its LH secretion (because it can see that enough testosterone is floating around, and it doesn't need to nudge the testicles to make more). Unfortunately, the brain also shuts down FSH, which is responsible for making sperm.

This results in two problems: The first is that when the testicles take a holiday, they may diminish in size, and smaller testicles can be a real bummer for some guys. More importantly, the snoozing testicles are also not manufacturing normal levels of sperm. This may be fine for men in their 40s and 50s who have no desire to add children to their flock. For younger males who want more children, testosterone supplementation can negatively affect their fertility.

HGH is a great solution for these younger men in that it mimics LH to stimulate the testicles to crank up their own natural production of testosterone while not impairing sperm production. We can give HGH alone or add HGH *with* testosterone replacement therapy to accommodate those concerned with the possibility of testicular shrinkage.

MONITORING YOUR TESTOSTERONE LEVELS

Once testosterone therapy gets underway, we usually obtain repeat lab values in two to three months. If necessary, the dose is adjusted, either up or down, based on the resolution of symptoms and the lab results. When symptoms of testosterone deficiency abate, and lab values are where they need to be, further testing can be conducted every six months to a year.

As mentioned previously, we monitor to ensure that both total and free testosterone levels are optimized. We make sure the testosterone is staying as testosterone and not being diverted to estrogen or DHT. We monitor PSA levels to confirm that the testosterone is having no effect on the prostate.

Another quirk with testosterone therapy is that it can rarely cause the blood to become overly concentrated. If that happens, you will need to donate a pint or two of blood to get levels back to normal before testosterone therapy can resume.

METHODS AND TIMING OF MONITORING

Testosterone therapy can be monitored using saliva, blood, or urine. Each method has advantages and disadvantages, although most practitioners use blood testing to monitor patients. Timing is everything! Depending on how the testosterone is administered, blood samples taken at the wrong time can give false information to the doctor. Timing recommendations are as follows:

Creams and gels

Apply these compounds the night *before* a morning blood draw. If creams or gels are used the same morning as a blood draw, the testosterone levels will appear artificially high. The draw should also be done in an area where you typically don't apply the cream or gel, since placing a needle through a patch of skin covered with cream gives false high results.

Injections

Those receiving injections once a week should have their lab test drawn on the fifth or sixth day after injection (just before the next injection). If they're using testosterone just underneath the skin twice a week, the lab should be drawn on the day before the next injection.

WHO CAN'T HAVE TESTOSTERONE REPLACEMENT THERAPY

Although testosterone therapy has not been demonstrated to cause prostate cancer, there is the possibility that it can feed an already active prostate cancer. For that reason, men with active prostate cancer do not qualify for this therapy. Other men who don't qualify include those with high hemoglobin levels (concentrated blood), patients with PSA levels greater than 4.0 (until they are cleared by a urologist), and anyone suffering from sleep apnea or severe cardiac, hepatic, or renal disease. Testosterone replacement therapy can potentially exacerbate all of these conditions.

Take this quiz and see if low testosterone may be a problem for you:

www.IntegrativeMedicineDallas/testosterone_quiz.com

CHAPTER 5

Optimizing Your Thyroid: Adding a Little Zip to Your Life

THE PROBLEM

Millions of patients, especially women, suffer from hypothyroidism (low thyroid levels) and are completely unaware of it. They just know they feel "crappy."

- They notice that they can't keep weight off the way they used to.
- Their energy levels are low, and they tend to "crash" every day around 3 p.m.
- They find themselves crawling, not springing, out of bed in the morning.
- They complain of always being cold, and they bug their spouses or co-workers to turn up the heat.
- Their memory is a little sketchy at times, and their concentration is not as focused as it used to be.
- Their fingernails get brittle, and their hair gets thin and

stringy.

• They generally feel that their battery is running low.

These complaints are often attributed to the demands of being a parent or a spouse, workplace stress, or the old standby of just getting older. Does this sound like you? This problem of hypothyroidism is *extremely* common, and the solution is elegant and simple. Yet so many people suffer needlessly. Simple awareness of the signs and symptoms of hypothyroidism is the first step.

WHAT MAKES YOUR THYROID GLAND GO CRAZY?

As we age there is a steady decline in our thyroid hormone levels. There are many reasons for this. Sometimes the brain quits stimulating the thyroid gland. Sometimes our diet is deficient in nutrients needed to make the hormone in the first place. Chronic stress, illness, and many medications can also take their toll on thyroid function.

Occasionally, the cells of our bodies can become resistant to the effects of thyroid hormone—something called thyroid resistance. Additionally, some of us develop autoimmune antibodies against the thyroid gland or thyroid hormone, impairing thyroid activity. Oh, and low thyroid levels can affect other hormones—and low or high hormones elsewhere can mess up the thyroid!

The problem can be very convoluted, confusing, circular, and complex to the uninitiated. Yet once the causes are teased out, the solutions are relatively straightforward. Patient awareness of common symptoms and vigilance on the part of the physician are the keys to success.

THE THYROID DEMOGRAPHIC

Low thyroid hormone levels, or hypothyroidism, are present

in one out of every seven adults. Women seem to be at greater risk for developing low thyroid hormone levels than men, although men are by no means excluded. Thyroid deficiency can occur at any age, yet it frequently raises its nasty head in the late 30s and early 40s. It often goes undetected in women as they approach menopause, since the symptoms of both conditions are often intertwined and similar.

WHAT DOES THYROID HORMONE DO ANYWAY?

The short answer is *a lot*! The thyroid gland is a little butterfly-shaped organ located in the middle of the neck. Thyroid hormone helps to regulate your body's metabolism. It also manages your energy levels and influences your body temperature (it sets your internal thermostat). It plays a role in increasing the breakdown of fat, resulting in weight loss and lower cholesterol. It has a role in protecting you from cardiovascular disease. Normal thyroid levels facilitate optimal brain function and help prevent cognitive impairment by improving memory and focus. Every cell of the body has thyroid hormone receptors on them, and thus, every cell in the body is negatively influenced when thyroid hormone doesn't show up for work.

THYROID HORMONE NUTS AND BOLTS

The brain produces a chemical which travels to the thyroid gland and tells it to make thyroid hormone. This chemical is called TSH (thyroid stimulating hormone). If thyroid levels get a little low, the brain makes more TSH to nudge the thyroid gland into making more hormones. If the thyroid gland doesn't or can't respond to its marching orders, the TSH levels remain elevated, continually trying to coax the thyroid gland to get with the program.

Once stimulated by TSH, a healthy thyroid gland produces

two "*flavors*" of thyroid hormone. T4 is the predominant hormone produced. T4 is essentially inactive and needs to be converted elsewhere in the body to the active form, called T3. The thyroid gland also produces a little T3 of its own. T4 and T3 ride around in the blood attached to little carrier proteins. Once they reach their destination, they *need to be converted,* and the inactive T4 is converted to active T3. Free T3 then enters the cell to perform its magic. It's the free T3 that is essentially driving your entire metabolic engine. That is why the amount of free T3 levels in your blood is the most important element in determining your overall thyroid function. TSH and T4 are also important, but to a lesser degree. (There are some instances when this simple pathway can get a bit convoluted, and we will discuss that shortly).

SYMPTOMS OF HYPOTHYROIDISM (LOW THYROID)

Since thyroid hormone affects every cell in the body, thyroid hormone deficiency causes lots of problems and can have several seemingly unrelated symptoms. They can be vague and nonspecific and confused with other problems. They can overlap with other issues that also need to be addressed. The list is long but very important. Symptoms include:
- dry skin, brittle nails
- hoarse voice
- thinning hair or hair loss
- cold hands and feet
- muscle fatigue, pain, and weakness
- poor memory and concentration
- heavy menstrual bleeding, worsening PMS, and infertility
- loss of sex drive
- severe menopausal symptoms such as hot flashes and mood swings

a fluid retention, swelling of hands and feet, puffy eyes
- low blood pressure and heart rate
- elevated cholesterol and triglycerides
- memory and concentration problems or brain fog
- fatigue, trouble getting out of bed in the morning
- loss or thinning of the outer third of your eyebrow
- trouble losing weight or recent weight gain
- depression, apathy, and anxiety
- constipation

DIAGNOSING THE PROBLEM

Many people who go to their doctor with these complaints and have their thyroid function evaluated are told that their thyroid is normal. Frequently, however, they are suffering from significant hypothyroidism. How can this be? Most physicians use TSH as their sole guide to determining whether or not a patient has a thyroid issue. For hypothyroidism, they are looking for a high TSH—made by the brain in response to low thyroid levels. But here is the problem. By only measuring TSH, over 80 percent of people with low thyroid are misdiagnosed!

It is possible (and fairly common) to have a normal TSH but have low thyroid hormone levels. Similarly, T4 and T3 levels can also be "normal" in people suffering from a hypothyroid condition.

What's going on here? The problem is that most physicians use the wrong tests to assess the thyroid. That is the way they were trained. They are searching for thyroid disease, not looking for optimal thyroid performance.

Unfortunately, you can be disease free yet still be suffering from several symptoms of low thyroid levels. This is a common mistake and the reason many patients suffer needlessly. This is an education issue for physicians, and many are slow to embrace this knowledge. Additionally, a TSH level is the only screening lab value that many insurance companies will cover. This is an example of how letting insurance companies dictate patient care is bad medicine.

Once again—what constitutes "normal?" Normal ranges used by laboratories are determined by taking the average lab values of a large number of very diverse people in terms of age, gender, ethnic and cultural background, diet, activity level, and the presence or absence of other illnesses. Common sense tells us that what is normal for an 80-year-old sedentary female may not be normal for a 27-year-old active, healthy male. Normal for your age does not translate into optimal for any age. In order to assess thyroid function properly, we need to know several things. We need to know how your adrenal glands are functioning and what kind of stress you are under. High stress causes high cortisol levels, which is well known to quash thyroid function. We know that estrogen dominance, experienced by many females suffering from PMS or during perimenopause, also adversely affects thyroid function. We need to ensure that critical elements such as selenium, iodine, zinc, and vitamin D are present in adequate amounts to support thyroid function. We need to know if gastrointestinal problems, which can cause chronic inflammation and trigger autoimmune disease of the thyroid gland, are an issue.

All of these things contribute to a broken thyroid and must be incorporated into the decision tree before an effective treatment plan can be devised.

OTHER THYROID BUG-A-BOOS
THE BRAIN AND TSH

The brain's ability to secrete TSH can be impaired for many reasons. A normal or low TSH level by no means insures good thyroid function. Sometimes the brain's ability to crank out enough TSH is broken, and like Scotty likes to say on Star Trek, "She's giving it all she's got."

The thyroid gland may require more motivation than it is receiving from the brain (TSH). In reality, it is responding appropriately to the weak signal it is receiving. Only by measuring free T4, free T3, reverse T3, and thyroid antibodies can we have a comprehensive snapshot of what the thyroid gland is really up to.

REVERSE T3—FRIEND AND FOE

Sometimes, conditions such as chronic stress, illness, fasting, and even certain medications can impair the conversion of T4 to T3 (the active form of thyroid). This results in low T3, and adding more T4 (Synthroid) obviously won't fix it.

Additionally, under times of psychological or physiologic stress, the body can put the brakes on the effects of thyroid hormone. This will protectively throttle down the metabolism by making something called reverse T3, instead of T3. Reverse T3 will snatch the receptor sites for thyroid hormone on the cells and won't let the all-important T3 into the cells to do its job.

So, although you may have normal free T4 and free T3 levels in your blood, elevated reverse T3 spoils the party by not letting T3 into the cell to do its work. This needs to be identified before thyroid hormone optimization can work. That is why giving just Synthroid, *which is straight T4*, as many practitioners do, can be ineffective. The T4 either can't convert to T3 (the good stuff), or makes reverse T3, which doesn't work.

DON'T FORGET THE IMMUNE SYSTEM

But wait! There's more. If anti-thyroid antibodies are floating around, the picture can get very complicated because the lab values for thyroid hormone may appear normal (or even elevated) even though your are, for all practical purposes, in a low-thyroid state. Your body can attack your own thyroid gland for many reasons, and it's not that uncommon. In my practice, I see antithyroid antibodies all the time.

WHAT DOES ALL THIS MEAN TO YOU?

It means that we must perform proper testing of thyroid function before we can come up with a good plan of action. A normal TSH level is of no value to us. We need to take a complete look at the effects of diet, nutritional status, hormone balance, and other illnesses or medications to nail down this diagnosis. At a minimum, this requires the following: TSH (we want this to be below 2, not the traditional 4.5), free T3, free T4, reverse T3, and anti-thyroid antibodies.

TREATING LOW THYROID

As mentioned, the traditional approach to treating hypothyroidism, when diagnosed, is usually with Synthroid (T4). We discussed earlier that straight T4 may not get to where it needs to be to improve thyroid hormone blood levels of T3 to relieve symptoms. Using a combination of both T4 and T3 (such as Armour thyroid) and specifically targeting free T3 levels is very effective in alleviating the symptoms of hypothyroidism. Sometimes we might even need to use straight T3 (jet fuel for the body!) for symptomatic relief if several of the T4 to T3 blocking mechanisms are in play.

Once the diagnosis is made and treatment begun, most patients begin to feel much better within two weeks. We usually retest blood levels within six to eight weeks and check symptoms to make dose adjustments. After that, retesting once or twice a year is sufficient.

CHAPTER 6

STRESS AND YOUR ADRENAL GLANDS: CHILL OUT AND LIVE LONGER

WHAT'S ALL THE STRESS ABOUT?

Stress! The pressure cooker between your ears that drives you crazy. Work, exams, the neighbor's cat, the neighbor *himself*! Your partner (in crime or in love), your boss, credit card bills, traffic, long lines, spelling mistakes—anything or everything can lead to stress. It's that overpowering feeling of fear and anxiety that drums in our heads, stealing our smiles and robbing us of our inner peace.

Stress can be quite limiting, as it can lead to guarded behavior, strained relationships, and an inability to complete tasks. Stress, as such, is not always to be maligned, as some amount of stress is good. Sometimes we need a fire lit underneath us to get the ball rolling. It is the level and duration of stress that is cause for worry.

To understand stress, we first need to understand the different types of stress.

TYPES OF STRESS

Routine stress is due to routine responsibilities like exams or work. These are everyday stressors and the constant whacks that keep our systems on their toes.

Sudden negative impact stress is caused when there is a drastic calamity in a person's life like a tornado, the death of a loved one, or the loss of a job.

Traumatic stress is caused when you are in danger and forced to flee or fight to stay alive. Some people undergo a condition called post-traumatic stress disorder after a traumatic event requiring therapy or counseling to help get over it.

In most instances, sudden negative impact stress and traumatic stress are unexpected, and it would be difficult to prepare yourself for them. But routine stress can snowball and mushroom into a monster that can chip away at your very core, eventually causing you to self-destruct.

We've all come to accept stress as a normal part of our lives, without realizing its considerable impact on our health. To understand the health implications of stress, let us first identify the symptoms of prolonged stress.

THE PICTURE OF STRESS

Here is a partial list of symptoms that chronic stress may cause:
- anxiety
- chronic allergies
- irritable bowel syndrome
- fatigue
- obesity
- depression

•brain fog

People differ considerably in how they deal with stress. While some people suffer from frequent headaches, others experience bowel irregularities. Though the symptoms encountered vary, the impact on our quality of life, and ultimately, our health, are the same.

MAGNITUDE OF THE PROBLEM

It is estimated that over 40 percent of all adults suffer from *chronic stress*, and over 75 percent of all visits to primary care physicians are in some way connected to the adverse health effects of stress. Stress has been directly linked to all the leading causes of death, including cardiovascular disease and cancer.

Chronic stress is everywhere and upends the quality of life for millions.

SOME JARRING FACTS ABOUT STRESS

According to the American Institute of Stress:

- Forty-three percent of all adults suffer adverse health effects due to stress-related complaints or disorders.
- Stress has been linked to leading causes of death, including heart disease, cancer, lung ailments, cirrhosis of the liver, and suicide.
- An estimated one million US workers are absent on any given workday due to stress-related complaints.
- Nearly half of all American workers suffer from symptoms of burnout.

According to the National Institute of Occupational Safety and Health:

- Forty percent of workers feel their job is very or extremely stressful.
- Twenty-five percent say their job is the number one stress-

or in their lives.

Where does all this stress come from and how do we generate it? Let's find out.

THE STRESS RESPONSE: A CRITICAL TOOL FOR SURVIVAL

The stress response is an ancient protective tool designed to get you out of a tight spot immediately! Imagine this: you visit the zoo, only to find out that you are now face to face with a lion that has escaped from its cage. There is no time to think or to wait for an escape route. You have to run, and fast, to stay alive. This sudden burst of energy and the drive to survive is fuelled by a stress response that increases the levels of the hormones cortisol and epinephrine helping you "get out of Dodge" as soon as possible!

The hormone cortisol, secreted by the adrenal glands, increases blood glucose levels during periods of acute stress in order to meet the immediate survival demands of the brain, heart, lungs, and muscles. In some cases, it even breaks down, or sacrifices, important proteins in the body to make even more blood glucose. Scientists E. H. Mathews and L. Liebenberg, in a study published in the journal *Stress Health* in October 2012, have pointed out that high levels of stress were found to increase blood glucose levels 2.2 times above normal levels.

This mechanism has been a lifesaver for thousands of years. This fight-or-flight response is seen today in our modern day zoos, also called the office. Though there are no lions, tigers, or bears, we live in a 24/7 over-connected, fast-paced, high-demand culture, where we have collectively forgotten how to relax. We are under constant pressure, either physically or mentally. Our old protector, the stress response, now works against us, because it is working overtime in situations for which it was never intended. The "on" button of our stress box is stuck, causing significant illness and disease in our society. In essence, our stress response is confused! Today, many things other than lions, tigers, and bears turn it on and keep it turned on far longer than it was designed for . . . and the consequences are killing us!

The most important stress hormone is called cortisol. Cortisol's ancient survival-based functions include:

- diverting the body's essential resources toward survival mode;
- increasing blood sugar, pulse, respiratory rate, and blood pressure (along with epinephrine);
- shutting down unnecessary functions like reproduction, immune systems, endocrine function, growth and repair, and anything else not needed to outrun lions (!);
- reducing stomach acid production and increasing the pace of food elimination in the intestinal tract (*We don't need to carry anything extra while outrunning lions!*); and,
- heightening your brain awareness and focus, so no sleep for you!

In short, cortisol turns off all non-essential systems that don't contribute to immediate survival in a threat scenario. It places them on hold, with the hope they can be switched back on soon IF survival indeed occurs.

Now that we know how our body responds to stress, let's look at possible sources of stress.

HITTING THE STRESS BUTTON

My patients are always surprised to learn of all the things that trigger stress . . .

- *Psychological stress*: job, spouse, kids, finances, psychological disorders (depression, anxiety, etc.), low self-esteem, and the state of the world (the international political situa-

tion, problems in your city or neighborhood)
- *Environmental stress*: chemical toxins, pollution, noise radiation, consumer products, medical procedures, radon, and cosmic rays
- *Food and water sources*: additives and preservatives, contamination, and highly processed artificial foods
- *Medication*: both prescription and over-the-counter drugs
- *Physiologic stress*: poor sleep, poor nutrition, illness, pain, inflammation, too much exercise, obesity, allergies, chronic infections, alcohol, tobacco, hormone imbalances, and severe climates

Stressors go beyond where you work and whom you are married to. Anything your body perceives as disrupting balance, whether internal or external, is a stressor.

Stress is defined as a real or perceived threat to your body. This can be physical or psychological. Psychological issues such as depression, anxiety, low socioeconomic status, divorce, loneliness, and unemployment can have profound physical effects on your health due to a prolonged stress response.

Stress is not limited by age, and even adolescents show symptoms of stress. For adolescents, however, as scientists K. Murray and colleagues discovered, body shape was the number one stressor! In this study, published in the journal *Stress Health* on July 30, 2013, 515 adolescents aged between 12 and 16 years were studied. The study showed that adolescents who had higher body dissatisfaction had greater stress levels due to peer pressure and poor self-esteem. Often the biggest stressors are not things, but people—and specifically, our thoughts about them. The *perception* aspect of chronic stress is very important and will be discussed later when we delve into fixing it.

If stress is a good thing, as it gets us out of trouble, then why are we so focused on reducing it? As mentioned earlier, it is the magnitude and duration of stress that is the problem. Let's find out what happens during extended periods of stress.

WHEN CHRONIC STRESS MAKES US SICK

Clearly, the adaptive stress response is beneficial in the short term. But what happens when the hormone cortisol, initially designed to protect us from imminent death, is secreted for longer periods?

THE ROLE OF CORTISOL

Cortisol is your body's primary wear and tear hormone. It is that hormone that fuels the escape from an assailant or enables us to fight off a threat. This wonder hormone can make glucose from almost anything, including bone, muscles, and other tissues if necessary. In an emergency, our body can and does devote all of its resources to the stress response for immediate survival.

When cortisol is persistently high, our body gets worn down. With chronic elevated cortisol levels, growth hormone levels fall, testosterone and progesterone levels fall, and thyroid function is disrupted. Our immune system, too, becomes suppressed. There is increased insulin resistance, and the resulting high blood sugar makes us fat. Our memory and ability to concentrate and focus begin to dwindle.

When cortisol is released into the bloodstream, you become less sensitive to leptin, a hormone that tells your brain you are full and to stop eating. It also makes you crave sugar, an evolutionary drive to consume calories to help face the dangers at hand.

When the body is fixed in the survival mode, constantly trying to protect itself from an alien threat, it fails to relax, with a drop in growth and development. It's analogous to driving a swanky, new sports car across hilly, bumpy roads with very little fuel in store. What's the need for speed when your tire is flat or your chassis is worn down or when your fuel tank is empty?

What's more, it's just not stress while at work that raises the salivary cortisol; even thinking about work and stressing over it can increase it! In a study published in the journal *Stress Health* in October 25, 2013, Croupley and several colleagues studied the effect of thinking about work on salivary cortisol levels. They found that when people thought about their day's work in the morning, it resulted in maximum cortisol secretion; conversely, those secretions were low late into the night. So Monday morning madness is not a myth.

The constant stress on the body has been implicated in a number of chronic degenerative diseases, which include:

- diabetes
- high blood pressure
- heart disease
- stroke
- cancers of all types
- infertility
- obesity
- metabolic syndrome
- inflammation
- mood disorders
- dementia
- osteoporosis
- irritable bowel syndrome

The extreme levels of stress we carry around today are an eye-opener to the kind of society that we have evolved into. Even when we are not in any real danger, we are stressed due to our complex psychology where we often stress about things that ultimately have very little impact on our physical safety.

High levels of stress are now the hallmark of prime jobs, resulting in more and more people feeling the need to be stressed to validate the importance of their work and their usefulness to the company. We live with chronic stress every day, caused by working too much, marital tension, lack of sleep, too much to do, and too little time in which to do it.

Ultimately, how we perceive and react to stress is vitally important in determining whether we will remain healthy. How we choose to manage stress puts us at risk of developing unhealthy coping behaviors such as smoking, overeating, or excessive alcohol consumption. Resorting to such habits causes even more damage to your health. In order to protect yourself from the adverse effects of stress, it is important to understand how chronic stress progresses.

RAMPING UP STRESS—THE THREE PHASES OF CHRONIC STRESS

Chronic stress progresses through three separate stages of severity. This is important because the treatment of chronic stress depends upon which stage you are in. Initially, a stressful event causes an increase in cortisol, which is a normal stress response and helps the body prepare for action or survive the "hit."

Eventually, with prolonged stress, DHEA (cortisol's support system) begins to fade, leaving unsupported, high cortisol levels. This is the state in which most people find themselves in the highly stressed society that we live in. This heightened state can last for decades, like a coiled spring waiting to explode. Eventually, if left unabated, the brain will try to protect itself from the relentless torture of high levels of cortisol by shutting down the adrenal glands.

Stage 1: The Alarm Reaction

This is the classic "fight or flight" reaction, also called "stressed and wired." The brain senses a threat and floods the body with both epinephrine and cortisol. Saliva tested at this stage would contain high levels of both these hormones. This stage is the reason the whole system was designed in the first place.

Stage 2: Resistance—Your Body Pushes Back

This is seen in a prolonged stress situation, also called "stressed and tired." Cortisol levels continue to hum along at high levels and begin having adverse effects on our health. Remember that elevated cortisol places everything important physiologically on hold. This includes normal maintenance and repair.

In this phase, the body starts to get tired of the whole situation, and DHEA levels start to drop. DHEA has many significant functions, the most important being to help keep the effects of cortisol in check (kind of like a chaperone). Testing in phase 2 reveals high cortisol levels and low DHEA.

Stage 3: Exhaustion—Throwing In the Towel

Exhaustion is also described as "stressed and depleted." During this stage, the whole system comes crashing down and the brain says, "Enough!" In an attempt to interrupt this seemingly endless destructive cycle, the brain just shuts the whole stress response machine down. This has classically been referred to as adrenal fatigue. In reality, the adrenal glands are working just fine, but the brain flips the off switch.

At this stage, all the body's systems are beat up and malfunctioning on many levels. Cortisol and DHEA are both in the basement, and the person has no stress response protection at all. This requires aggressive intervention by a knowledgeable physician to get back on track. Since the levels of cortisol soar when the body is under stress, let's look more closely at what the hormone actually does to the body.

HIGH CORTISOL VS. LOW CORTISOL—THE DIFFERENCES AND SIMILARITIES

HIGH CORTISOL (STAGE 1 AND 2)

Although the initial stages of the stress response are intended to promote survival, chronic exposure to stressors can have adverse effects on every organ system in the body. These organ systems eventually succumb to the wear and tear of cortisol gone awry. The immune system is one of the primary systems affected. This translates into an increased susceptibility to infection and cancer.

As stated earlier, prolonged stress inhibits the nonessential functions of growth, repair, and reproduction. Therefore, growth hormone, thyroid hormone, testosterone, estrogen, and progesterone are all affected by chronic stress.

Elevated cortisol also affects insulin release and glucose regulation. Chronically elevated cortisol levels increase insulin. Chronically elevated insulin leads to insulin resistance and obesity. This sets up a chain reaction for the eventual development of diabetes, high cholesterol, cardiovascular disease, and hypertension. In fact, researchers have clearly shown that high cortisol states increase the risk of mortality by three times. Life expectancy decreases by several years.

Other conditions related to chronically elevated cortisol levels include anorexia nervosa, obsessive-compulsive disorder, panic disorder, chronic alcoholism, excessive exercising, and depression.

SYMPTOMS OF ELEVATED CORTISOL

Symptoms include irritability, anxiety, fatigue, low energy (especially in the morning), night sweats, hot flashes, sleep disturbance, sugar cravings, weight gain, confusion and poor mental function and focus, depression, memory loss, and low libido.

LOW CORTISOL: PHASE III STRESS (ADRENAL FATIGUE)

Eventually, the brain will attempt to protect the body from the ravages of over-the-top cortisol levels. It takes charge and shuts down the adrenal glands, plunging the body into a low-cortisol state, which is commonly called adrenal fatigue.

Low cortisol has been found in 25 percent of patients with these stress-related bodily disorders:

- chronic fatigue syndrome
- fibromyalgia
- irritable bowel syndrome
- chronic pain
- atypical depression

Patients with low cortisol or adrenal fatigue typically suffer from chronic fatigue, impaired cognition, sleep disturbances, anorexia, and depression. The low cortisol states of adrenal fatigue may result in an overactive immune system. This increases susceptibility to a variety of inflammatory diseases including autoimmune disease, malignancy, chronic pain syndromes, and fibromyalgia. Other conditions linked to low cortisol include hypothyroidism, rheumatoid arthritis, premenstrual syndrome, and early menopause.

SYMPTOMS OF LOW CORTISOL

The onset of adrenal fatigue is often insidious, and many of the signs and symptoms are vague and confusing. Patients may complain of low-grade fever, easy fatigability, muscle aches, weight loss, and muscle weakness. Some complain of abdominal pain, nausea and vomiting, and low blood sugar. In fact, the three most common complaints of people who have adrenal fatigue are a high sensitivity to stress, chronic fatigue, and chronic pain.

Other common symptoms include:

- *General*: fatigue, fever, weakness, muscle pain, joint pain, sore throat, headaches, dizziness upon standing, and chronic pain
- *Gastrointestinal*: lack of appetite, nausea, vomiting, diarrhea, and abdominal pain
- *Psychiatric*: depression, apathy, irritability, sleep disturbances, difficulty concentrating, difficulty with memory, confusion, stress sensitivity
- *Cardiovascular*: increased heart rate, dehydration, and low blood pressure

As these symptoms are similar to those in other medical conditions, patients with low cortisol often go undiagnosed or are simply diagnosed with chronic fatigue syndrome or depression. Another disturbing effect of low cortisol levels in the body is the onset of autoimmune disease. Let's read on to find out why.

STRESS AND AUTOIMMUNE DISEASE

In the face of low cortisol, the pro-inflammatory side of your immune system is no longer under the suppressive influence of cortisol. The parent is no longer around to control the child. Unsupervised, immune processes can go unchecked, causing destruction of your tissues in the form of autoimmune diseases.

The following autoimmune diseases have been associated with low cortisol:

- rheumatoid arthritis
- dermatitis
- type I diabetes
- multiple sclerosis
- Hashimotos thyroiditis

MAKING THE DIAGNOSIS

Doctors don't traditionally receive a great deal of training in the topic of stress during medical school. As mentioned, the three stages of chronic stress are stressed and wired, stressed and tired, and stressed and depleted. They can be diagnosed by a skilled examiner through a comprehensive history and physical examination. The best test to confirm the diagnosis and stage is a 24-hour saliva test to measure both cortisol and DHEA.

LIFESTYLE CHANGES TO OUTSMART STRESS

A whopping 50 percent of Americans take prescription drugs to suppress and disguise symptoms of stress, which is a real problem if you consider the side effects and drug dependency. Moreover, focusing merely on the symptoms will not help identify the stressor, so on and on the problem goes.

One antidote is to tap into your spiritual side. This does not mean diving headlong into something new and alien but gently easing yourself into certain aspects of spirituality that have appealed to you in the past. This means different things to different people. Research has shown that people who identify with a higher power or have a religious affiliation enjoy less stress, better health, and a longer lifespan.

Your diet also has a profound impact on your level of stress. The more processed, fried, and artificially colored the food you eat, the more the stress on your system. Of course, eating right does come with a huge side effect, a flat stomach!

Get enough sleep. The whole point is to wake up feeling well rested and happy. Be selfish and do whatever you need to for a good night's sleep. Choose thick curtains for the window. Soundproof your room, or if you have a noisy spouse, use earplugs (or sleep alone, if your marriage will allow!). If you have ever watched a 5-year-old after the kid has eaten a sucker, you will never eat sugar-rich food before bed. It will give you a sugar high that will keep you awake for hours, so stay away.

Meditate and learn to relax! Don't worry, be happy! Some people view relaxation as a task for the lazy, as all you do is sit around and sleep. Well, sometimes, that's all we need to get our batteries charged. In terms of stress management, it is highly therapeutic. Our bodies and brains need to decompress in order to work at optimal levels.

Exercise has been proven to be a great modifier of stress. Besides the obvious health benefits it serves as a useful 'outlet' for frustrations and shifts your thinking away from your worries and concerns.

Seek out some sort of social affiliation or support. It is always more stressful in most things going it alone. Be part of a group with a common cause or agenda. Support and social affiliation can come in the form of family, community or special interest groups.

Apart from these changes to your lifestyle, there are also certain supplements that can get your stress under control.

ADAPTOGENS

Adaptogens are compounds that increase your ability to adapt to and avoid damage from stressors. Adaptogens will help tone you down.

These are some adaptogens:
• ashwaganda

- rhodiola rosea
- Korean ginseng
- licorice
- cordyceps

VITAMINS, MINERALS, AND SUPPLEMENTS

Stress depletes your body of several vitamins and minerals that need to be replaced. Several supplements can help calm the effects of elevated cortisol on your brain.

Vitamin C: Your adrenal glands contain the highest concentration of vitamin C in your body. Chronic stress can lead to depletion of adrenal vitamin C stores.

Magnesium: Magnesium can be calming and help to correct anxiety and depression. Foods rich in magnesium are almonds, soybeans, cashews, spinach, and halibut.

B vitamins: Bs help to prevent high cortisol levels and improve cortisol balance.

Theanine: This is present in green tea and helps produce calming waves in your brain. It counteracts the stimulating effects of caffeine and prevents cortisol levels from getting too high when you're in high stress situations. Theanine is essentially nature's form of Xanax. Theanine does not have any side effects.

Phosphatidylserine: This prevents surges in cortisol, causes a decrease in post-exercise cortisol levels, and raises the levels of neurotransmitters, such as dopamine, thereby improving mood. It may prevent chronic, stress-induced memory loss.

DHEA: The DHEA and cortisol balance is very important. With high cortisol, DHEA supplementation can help to bring cortisol levels down and protect the brain and other tissues from its damaging effects.

GABA: GABA helps relieve anxiety and promotes relaxation and sleep.

Melatonin: Melatonin maintains normal circadian sleep cycles.

COPING WITH STRESS

One key to beating stress is to strive to be happy and optimistic. When you enjoy what you do and love it like nothing else, then you will love getting back to it again. Cultivate a sense of satisfaction and a general optimism that extends beyond work; this will help fight the blues. Y. Chang and H. G. Chan published a study on the effects of optimism on stress in the *Journal of Nursing Management* in its September 2013 issue. Three hundred fourteen staff nurses participated included in a study which assessed their levels of optimism and stress. Nurses who had an optimistic attitude enjoyed their work. and subsequently, had lower levels of stress. So pick yourself up, look into the mirror, and tell yourself you love your job—or choose a profession you love!

Be confident; this will go a long way in staving off peer pressure. Everybody is special, and it's all about finding out what's special about you and flaunting that. When you control your emotions like anger, you have a better control over your stress levels.

Remember, yesterday is history, tomorrow is a mystery — all we have for sure is today. Remain mindful and in the present when you can. Remember the saying recited in Alcoholics Anonymous meetings all over the world:

> God grant me the serenity
> to accept the things I cannot change;
> courage to change the things I can;
> and wisdom to know the difference

Don't let your psychology be the lion that perpetually chases you—constantly igniting the fight or flight machine in your head. Reframe what's important in the big picture. Slow down, relax, and take time to smell the roses.

Take this quiz to see if adrenal stress is a problem for you: www.IntegrativeMedicineDallas/adrenalstress_quiz.com

CHAPTER 7

NUTRITIONAL ARMAGEDDON: DEFENSIVE EATING FOR HEALTHY AGING

The food you choose will determine the state and health of your life. The key is, each day it's a choice. Food is medicine and you can heal your body by focusing on healthy choices.

Understanding one simple fact will determine ultimate success in staying healthy. Proper nutrition, as boring as that may sound, is unequivocally the most important part of any effort to be your best and prevent chronic disease. Period.

Hormone optimization, exercise, stress management, and "clean living" will all fail if you are not eating the right foods. It's just that simple. I can't say this strongly enough. This simple fact has huge implications and needs to really sink in! Look around you, and observe what happens when this fundamental principle is ignored. Welcome to modern Western culture.

OUR CURRENT FOOD LANDSCAPE

We live in a world where processed, high fat, sugar-laden foods are everywhere. Billions of dollars are spent each year marketing these foods to us and our children in increasingly creative ways. We live in a high stress, time-crunched society where convenience and expediency channel our behavior. The nostalgic Norman Rockwell home-cooked meal shared at the dining table—enjoying the company of family, and discussing life—is now the exception rather than the rule.

We now have ready access to a plethora of quick, inexpensive, and tasty food alternatives. They are methodically engineered by PhD food scientists to romance our brain cravings for sugar, fat, and salt. Our genetically modified crops are sprayed with toxic pesticides. The meat we consume is laced with antibiotics and hormones. For almost 200,000 years, these artificial foods didn't exist. Then, in a flash, they were everywhere. Industrialized food! Genetically speaking, our bodies are in a state of shock. Unfortunately, these toxic food imposters are all that most of us have ready access to.

HOW YOUR ANCIENT WIRING MAKES YOU FAT AND UNHEALTHY

Historically, famine was a universal certainty in all cultures. It was not a matter of *if* but *when* famine would strike. Throughout most of human history, food has been scarce. All food consumed was allocated very efficiently. Our ancient metabolic wiring was designed to maximize our survival potential.

Our metabolism is very efficient in scrounging calories from our diet and storing them for the day when famine would certainly rear its ugly head. Concurrently, our brain was programmed to crave and consume high calorie foods when available and lock them up in a storage bin that is difficult to access in the form of fat. Carbohydrates consumed were complex carbohydrates with a low glycemic index (slow release of sugar into our bloodstream). Since our metabolic blueprint is designed for calorie conservation, accumulated fat is surrendered very begrudgingly unless we are starving. Until relatively recently, these physiologic pathways were critical for ultimate survival.

In modern Western society, famine is no longer a player in our daily existence. However, our metabolic wiring remains unchanged. This wiring still expects famine to be a certainty, and our metabolic software obediently prepares for that eventuality. It is unaware that food is now abundant and that there is a fast food restaurant or convenience store on every corner.

Throughout most of human history, there was never a survival advantage to develop systems to curb consumption of high sugar or high-fat foods. On the contrary, we are driven by our DNA to get as much of it where and when we can. Our brain still motivates (*almost commands*) us to consume such food when available. A system of "food brakes" never developed.

Fast forward to today. We live in a sea of unprecedented abundance. Such abundance of calorie-rich foods requires our higher thinking centers to wrestle with our primal consumption instinctsto tell us that enough is enough. Clever marketers dangle fat, sugar, and salt at our senses everywhere we turn. They know how intensely our primal buttons are wired and intend to profit from that knowledge.

So, how is that working for us? Simple observation confirms that too many of us have lost that battle. Research has shown that food cravings light up the same addictive centers in our brain as those addicted to sex, drugs, and alcohol. And, as with all addictions, research also shows that the more you get, the more you want. Look around and observe that we want and want and can't stop.

Some pharmaceutical companies realize the similarities between food cravings and drug addiction physiology and are
even tampering with medications similar to those used in treating drug addiction to help curb overeating and food cravings.
The mechanism of abuse seems to be the same—whether it's
food or heroin.

WE ARE SURROUNDED BY ENABLERS

It is fascinating to observe how our biological programming
feeds cultural trends. The hit movies *Supersize Me* and *Fast
Food Nation*, as well as the hit documentary Food Inc., paint a
dismal portrait of our society's eating habits.

- One in four Americans visits a fast food restaurant every
  day.
- Over 40 percent of American meals are eaten outside of
  the home.
- McDonald's sees more than 46 million people a day. That is
  more than the entire population of Spain.
- French fries are the most eaten vegetable in America.
- One in three children born in the year 2000 will develop
  diabetes.
- Obesity will surpass smoking as the leading cause of preventable death in the United States.

Surprisingly, several revered organizations such as the
American Heart Association and the American Diabetic Association have contributed to this conundrum. Incorrect scientific assumptions from the late 1950s led to the establishment of
national dietary guidelines in the 1970s, which recommended
minimizing fat in our diet. This spawned an era of "fat phobia."

The United States Department of Health then recommended
that dietary fat be replaced with starchy carbohydrates such as
cereals, bread, rice, and pasta—the well-known but totally con-

fused Food Pyramid. The consequences of adopting these recommendations have been disastrous. Since then we've noticed a huge upward swing in average body weight. Over the past thirty years, the obesity rate has doubled. Among children, obesity has tripled. The incidence of adult onset diabetes (type II diabetes) has risen alarmingly, as have all obesity-related diseases.

It's interesting to note that people immigrating to the United States from countries that traditionally have a low incidence of cardiovascular disease and diabetes assume American disease rates upon adopting our diet high in refined carbohydrates (based on the standard American diet).

SUGAR AND INSULIN—THEIR TOXIC DANCE

The increased consumption of the newly abundant high carbohydrate foods has had a profound impact on sugar levels in our bloodstream. By eating the standard American diet, wide daily fluctuations in our average blood sugar has become the rule, rather than the exception.

Insulin is the hormone that opens the doors into our cells, allowing sugar to pass through and be burned as fuel. High blood sugar requires lots of insulin working overtime to stuff it into cells. Excess sugar needs to go somewhere, and insulin will store it as body fat and blood fat (triglycerides) for a rainy day.

Over time, these high insulin levels become ineffective because our cells start to ignore insulin, resulting in insulin resistance. When cells ignore insulin, sugar can't get to where it needs to go and starts to rise in the bloodstream. The pancreas fights back by making more insulin, which causes more insulin resistance. That results in insulin and blood sugar levels creeping up over time.

The body is now out of balance. High insulin and high blood sugar are both toxic and start all kinds of problems. Obesity and diabetes are the biggies; they are directly responsible for the majority of chronic health problems seen today, including heart disease, autoimmune disease, vascular disease, and dementia.

IT'S ALL BETWEEN THE EARS

Fortunately, as human beings, we have higher brain centers that can override our primal urges to consume the high calorie foods that constantly serenade us. Exercising this cognitive force can be difficult at best and demands an understanding of our ancient nutritional biology. Only when we understand our primal urges in the presence of plenty can we defeat them. Knowledge of our innate and irresistible tendencies arms us with cerebral ammunition to resist them and think our way to responsible eating, and thus, optimal health. Essentially, we need to outsmart ourselves.

A PRACTICAL REALISTIC APPROACH TO EATING SMART: IT'S NOT ABOUT STARVING!

In a nutshell: consume healthy, balanced, real foods. Don't worry about attaining a target weight, as is commonly recommended. The goal is to reduce body fat to a healthy level by eliminating key offenders to the battle of the bulge and to promote the right foods to prevent the chronic diseases that make us miserable in our 'mature' years.

I don't advocate a certain diet, since most diets are unsustainable and ultimately fail. A starvation diet, using the old, unenlightened, and incorrect "calories in versus calories out" equation, will never work over the long term. It ignores our physiology. Instead, it's best to align your eating behaviors with your ancient metabolic blueprint in a way that is sustainable with minimal pain. It comes down to what and how you eat—not how much you eat.

When combined with nutritional supplements, regular exercise, stress management, and bioidentical hormones when needed, you can be very successful in preventing or reversing obesity and stopping the progression of chronic disease in its tracks. Food is a powerful drug—eat the right stuff and your body will fall in line with its natural biology.

Having said that, it is important to remember that you can't ignore calories altogether. I don't mean to imply that you can eat 4,000 calories a day of good food and remain healthy. Eating 800 calories daily is also a terrible idea. What you need to understand is that the type of calories you consume and the percentage of calories obtained from good fat, protein, and carbohydrates is far more important than how much you eat. Given the right mix, your body will do the rest.

STUFF WE MEASURE
Metabolism

Let's start by determining a *ballpark idea* of how many calories you should consume each day. This number is based on your estimated basal metabolic rate (*BMR*), combined with the number of calories needed to maintain your particular activity level. Again, we don't advocate that you become a calorie counter, but getting an idea of your energy requirements is helpful.

BMR

Your basal metabolic rate makes up around 65 percent of your caloric requirements. This is the number of calories you burn when just sitting around quietly doing nothing but staring at the wall. These calories serve as energy for such activities as breathing, thinking, supplying your beating heart with energy, and maintaining body temperature.

Your basal metabolic rate is not static but is affected by several factors including age, weight, gender, environmental temperature, stress, concurrent illness, and diet. I won't bore you with the details of how this number is derived. Several resources are available free on the Internet to easily calculate your particular BMR.

Calories Needed to Fuel Your Individual Activity Level

This number is also easily attained from several free websites, including www.nutristrategy.com/activitylist.htm and *www.healthyweightforum.org/eng/calorie-calculator.asp.* Calculating the calories needed to sustain your average activity level plus your BMR will give you a good idea of your caloric requirements. Try your best to keep your calorie intake at this level and no higher. There is no need (in fact, it can be counterproductive) to cut calories significantly below your daily requirements. Your metabolism will simply slow down and make you miserable (low energy, foggy thinking, irritability, anxiety, and hunger).

Body Fat Percentage

In my opinion, this is the most important measurement needed to determine where you are and where you need to be to achieve optimum health. A DEXA scan is the most accurate method available. This machine uses very low-level X-rays to precisely calculate the percentage of your body that is fat. It also measure lean body mass.

Machines that measure bioelectrical impedance such as the Tanita scale (www.tanita.com) are also good and readily available for home use. This device is less accurate but still gives a pretty good idea of your body fat composition. Skinfold measurements are a down and dirty method using calipers, which measure skinfold thickness at various points on the body. This method has a high potential for inaccuracies but is a good way to spitball where you are. Healthy males should have a body fat percentage of under 20 percent and females a fat percentage of under 30 percent.

STACKING THE DECK: CRITICAL THINGS YOU NEED TO KNOW FOR SUCCESS

HOW TO EAT

It's critical to start out with the right mindset. You will need to change how you view food. Appreciate the fact that nutrition is the singular most important determinant of your health. View food as a valuable tool that serves you, rather than enslaves you. Realize that your body is an incredible metabolic machine requiring test-grade fuel to help it run smoothly and efficiently. Understand that food is the most powerful drug you consistently put into your body and even contains information that speaks to your DNA, giving it guidance and instruction (an interesting science called nutrigenomics).

The old view, one still held by many, is that calories are the problem, and all we have to do is eat less food and exercise more to avoid being fat. News flash!! Calories *in* DON'T equal calories *out*! It's not a two-way street. Once captured, your body will cling to stored calories with devotion and zest. Remember: it thinks famine is coming someday.

There is no running an extra mile to burn off that extra slice of pizza. It just doesn't work that way. You need to realize that all calories are not created equal, and the *type* of calories you consume is far more important than the *number*.

I want to re-emphasize that we discourage dieting. Most diets entail some form of calorie restriction. When you restrict calories, your body outsmarts you and simply dials down your metabolic engine to an idle. It can out-wait you!! Instead, I am going to help you establish new habits to replace bad habits. I want you eat good food in a more organized way—and perhaps a little less. (It's that addiction thing—more is better!!) Here are some important tips:

1. Never, ever skip meals. Skipping meals, especially breakfast, just slows down your metabolism. Your body says, "OK, you're not going to feed me? No, problem. I'll just turn down the furnace." Calories burn slower, and this defeats your goal. It also fires up your primitive brain to turn on your hunger and discomfort buttons, pushing you to binge on high calorie foods. (You can't win. Really. You have thousands of years of metabolic systems development against little ole' you.)

   When you're out and about, carry a small bag of nuts, low carb fruit, protein powder, or a protein bar to rescue you from cravings throughout the day and keep your engine stoked between meals so that is doesn't throttle down to an idle.

2. Always ensure that your meals are a balanced mix of protein, carbohydrates, and healthy fats. You may need professional guidance to determine what that balance is. There are even genetic tests available that can tell you the best mix for you.

3. Don't inhale your food. Eat slowly. Follow the Japanese tradition of putting down your fork when you are 80 percent full. Remember that it takes time for the signals from your stomach and blood sugar to reach your brain and tell you that you've had enough.

4. Make meals a communal event when possible. Avoid eating in your car, at your desk or in front of the television set. Never eat meals on the run. Savor your eating experience.

5. Hang out with people who share your nutritional and

lifestyle goals. Having overweight friends increases your chances of being overweight yourself by 57 percent according to a report in the *New England Journal of Medicine*. Hanging out with drinkers makes you more inclined to drink too much as well.

6. Remember your blood sugar. Think about the affect a food has on your blood sugar and the chain reaction of bad events and the results from sugar spikes. Strive to keep your blood sugar relatively constant and avoid having it ping all over the map.

7. Avoid emotional eating. Don't eat when you're bored, angry, stressed, or depressed. Eat only when you're hungry. In fact, when you feel like snacking, make a point to ask yourself, "Am I really hungry?"

8. Don't be a calorie counter. Always remember that counting calories is far less important than monitoring the type of foods that you eat.

   Remember that good nutrition involves conscious effort. Get rid of reflex behavior. Celebrate that you are an evolved creature who can exercise command over the universe through the power of choice. These choices fall within the spectrum of worse choice, better choice, and best choice.

9. Always shop along the perimeter of the supermarket. That is where the real food lives (real food needs refrigeration). The inner aisles are occupied by foods that are highly processed in order to be packaged, facilitating a long shelf life. If you can place a food item in your pantry for six months and bacteria won't touch it, then you probably shouldn't eat it either. Real food rots. Don't eat immortal food.

10. At home, clear the pantry and refrigerator of all processed, high fat, high carbohydrate foods. Try to have alcohol not so readily available, and make it so you have to

leave the house to get a drink.

11. Get the rest of your family on-board. This can be difficult when you're the lone voice of reason in the forest. There is strength in numbers. It DOES take a village.

WHAT TO EAT

The typical scenario goes something like this:

The average person will eat a high calorie breakfast consisting of pancakes, orange juice, toast or bagel, high sugar fruits, or cereal. Other people just don't have time for breakfast and skip it altogether. Both behaviors result in a blood sugar crash around ten o'clock in the morning. Around this time, you may get a little irritable, your energy may drop, and the hunger button gets turned on. This is where most of us will grab a candy bar or a snack out of the vending machine (chips) for a little extra boost.

Lunch is usually taken on the fly at your desk or at a nearby fast food establishment. Your blood sugar will soar and then crash around 3 p.m., resulting in another trip to the vending machine or a foray into your desk drawer for another high carbohydrate yummy. This boost will hold you over until dinner, where you'll consume the standard American diet of pasta, bread (hamburgers, pizza, and tacos), potatoes, or rice . . . all finished off with a glorious desert. That will get you through until around 8 or 9 p.m., when many people get the late-night munchies.

Then it's off to the fridge or pantry for a yummy treat (we seldom snack on broccoli). This final sugar assault of the day makes sleeping more difficult and sets you up for the early-morning crash. And on and on we go.

The net result is a blood sugar roller coaster, with insulin trying to keep up by packaging all that extra sugar into efficient little fat compartments to prepare you, once again, for the famine that is just over the horizon.

Let me suggest a better way. It is important to design your meals for a balanced mix of carbohydrate, protein, and fat. This may sound rather technical and even daunting but is actually quite easy to do. Simply stated, by the end of the day you want your calorie spread to be like this:

- carbohydrate: 40 to 45 percent
- protein: 30 to 35 percent
- healthy fats: 20 -percent

CARBOHYDRATES

All carbohydrates are not created equal. We need to be careful which ones we eat.

SIMPLE CARBS

Simple carbohydrates are primarily sugars. They are found in candy, cakes, cookies, sodas, alcohol, and fruit juices. These carbohydrates are digested quickly and transform almost immediately into blood sugar. This blood sugar spike wakes up insulin, which very efficiently stores this excess sugar as fat.

Simple carbohydrates really have nothing of value nutritional to offer and are referred to as empty calories. They generally contain no vitamins, minerals, fiber, or any other important nutritional elements. There are some foods containing simple carbohydrates that possess some nutritional benefit. Fruits, milk, yogurt, and other dairy products are great examples. We recommend no more than 10 percent of your total carbohydrate intake come from these sources.

Simple carbohydrates sneak into your diet in nefarious ways. Processed foods frequently have simple sugars added to them for flavor. If you read labels, you will find these sugars listed as honey, molasses, cornstarch, maltose, laevulose, fructose, sucrose, lactose, and high fructose corn syrup.

COMPLEX CARBS

Complex carbohydrates come in two varieties: starchy and fibrous. Starchy complex carbohydrates include grains such as cereals and bread, potatoes, white rice, pastas, and crackers. Although starchy carbohydrates have some nutritional value, they convert readily and quickly to blood glucose and should be consumed sparingly and occasionally.

Fibrous complex carbohydrates are found primarily in vegetables, nuts, and legumes. These foods are packed with nutrients, especially the vegetables. They are critical elements in our diet. Their fibrous construction results in a slow release of the sugars they contain, which keeps the blood sugar levels beneath the insulin radar.

Fruits are also complex fibrous carbohydrate sources. One or two pieces of fruit a day is fine. It is important to remember that not all fruits are created equal, either. Some, such as melons, bananas, mangoes, and pineapples, have a high glycemic index (meaning they raise your blood sugar quickly). You should also avoid all dried fruits (as seen in trail mixes), because the drying process concentrates the sugars. Plums, apples, cherries, berries, and oranges are great examples of low glycemic index fruits and are preferred if you are going to eat fruit.

FATS

Fats are found everywhere in our food supply. They can be found in meat, dairy products, oils, olives, nuts, and vegetables, just to name a few. There are two main types of fats: saturated and unsaturated (these terms relate to their chemistry and explain how the hydrogen atoms are arranged, just in case you ever wondered). In general, unsaturated fats are healthier and are preferred.

Saturated fats are sometimes called "bad fats." For the most part, they are not healthy and can contribute to cardiovascular disease. The main sources of saturated fats come from animal products such as fatty red meat and whole milk dairy products (always try to eat lean meats and low-fat dairy products). There are also plant-based sources of saturated fat, primarily from the following oils: corn, sunflower, safflower, grape seed, and cottonseed. Many of our most beloved foods contain high levels of saturated fats. This includes fried foods such as fried chicken and French fries, pizza, and most baked goods.

Unsaturated fats are "good fats." They come in two forms: Monosaturated and polyunsaturated. The majority of your fat intake should come from foods containing these fats. They include nut butters, fish, avocado, nuts, and healthy oils (extra virgin olive oil, canola, avocado, walnut, coconut, flaxseed, macadamia nut, and sesame).

Anyone who reads the newspapers has heard about *trans fats*. These are unsaturated fats that, due to processing, morph into a configuration not seen in nature. It is common knowledge that these fats are terrible for your health. You will find these dangerous fats in margarine, packaged foods, frozen foods, store-bought soups, and fast food. Avoid these like the plague.

Moderate amounts of healthy fat in your diet are critical for health. This fact is hard to accept by our current fat-phobic culture. Remember that despite what we have been told all these years, eating fat doesn't make you fat. We just need to be smart and choose the right kinds of fat.

PROTEIN

Proteins are part of every cell, tissue, and organ in our body. It is our raw construction material, like bricks are for a building. Unlike glucose, proteins cannot be readily stored in the body. Proteins must be consumed with every meal to maintain an optimal rate of growth and repair. If you become deficient in protein, your body will break down muscle tissue to get it. Good sources of protein include lean red meat, poultry, fish, whey protein powders, low-fat milk, and dairy products.

A SPECIAL NOTE ABOUT ALCOHOL

Most experts agree that alcohol is a diet wrecker and contributes significantly to being overweight. After all, alcohol constitutes another form of a simple carbohydrate and elevates your blood sugar rapidly. Although a valuable social lubricant, it is an empty carb nutritionally that needlessly adds unnecessary calories to the bottom line.

Alcohol also ramps up your appetite, and individuals tend to overeat when alcohol is served with a meal according to two studies published in the *American Journal of Clinical Nutrition*. Alcohol also induces the liver to produce more fatty acid and is a major cause in elevated blood triglycerides (blood fat).

Surprisingly, many people don't realize just how much alcohol they consume. The caloric contribution from alcohol consumption sneaks up on them over time. One drink a day represents 33,600 calories per year. Two drinks a day adds up to a whopping 67,000 calories per year. Did you know that 3,500 calories is equal to one pound of fat?

The specter of going the rest of your life without consuming alcohol is disturbing for most people. The good news is that two or three alcoholic drinks a week is acceptable while maintaining a healthy lifestyle. These intermittent hits to your metabolism are well tolerated. However, until you are close to your ideal body weight and are engaged in a good nutrition and exercise program, the more you abstain from alcohol, the better. Don't worry, it shouldn't take too long for you to get on the healthy track and start enjoying alcohol again responsibly.

WHEN TO EAT

Enjoy six small meals a day, eating every three hours. This keeps your blood sugar relatively stable and avoids sugar dips between meals that lead to snacking and binging. Remember, blood sugar excesses throughout the day are quickly turned to fat, while blood sugar dips (skipping meals) put the brakes on your metabolism, slowing your calorie burning machinery. Here is a good way to break up your eating day:

- breakfast
- midmorning snack
- lunch
- midafternoon snack
- dinner
- evening snack

Small, frequent meals throughout the day evenly fuel your metabolism and avoid energy peaks and valleys. A steadily churning metabolism running in high gear helps keep body fat in check.

BREAKFAST

After fasting all night, bread is critical to start your metabolic engine for the day and to keep it humming. A good breakfast, like all of your meals, should provide a balance of all three primary energy sources (carbohydrates, proteins, and fats). Examples of a healthy breakfast include:

- a three-egg omelet, with two strips of turkey bacon and some blueberries; or
- a whey-protein shake. These shakes can be quite yummy and usually come in flavors of chocolate, vanilla, or straw-

berry. They take less than five minutes to prepare. They are best when placed in a blender with a few ice cubes to give them a milkshake-like texture. You can also include fruit or cocoa powder in your whey-protein shake. Snazz it up a little bit!

LUNCH AND DINNER

We recommend a Mediterranean diet which emphasizes healthy fats like olive oil, steamed or grilled vegetables in a natural state, along with portions of fish (salmon), grilled poultry (chicken or turkey), or small amounts of lean red meat.

Several internationally renowned nutritional experts as well as the Mayo Clinic have endorsed the Mediterranean diet as the best diet for reducing insulin resistance and diabetes, inflammatory conditions, high cholesterol, high blood pressure, heart disease, and colon cancer. The Mediterranean diet includes:

- vegetables and fruit
- nuts, seeds, and beans
- healthy oils, such as olive oils
- lean meats, such as turkey or chicken
- lean red meat twice a week
- fish, especially tuna and salmon
- eggs

This diet avoids most breads, pastas, crackers, potatoes, and creamy or cheesy sauces. (You know, all the stuff we love.)

The Internet is a rich resource containing multiple recipes for a delicious assortment of meals as part of a modified Mediterranean diet program.

SNACKS

Snacks are very important. They keep your blood sugar stable throughout the day and keep your metabolic engine humming along at full throttle. Remember, when your blood sugar is low between meals, your metabolism slows down and your energy levels drop. Intermittent snacks prevent this from happening.

The same rules apply for snacks as they do for all of your meals. They should contain some protein and a complex carbohydrate. Unhealthy snacks (the average American snack such as cookies, crackers, potato chips, soft drinks, etc.) are laced with simple carbohydrates; they ultimately defeat everything you are trying to accomplish. Healthy snacks include:

- a meal replacement protein shake or protein bar.
- vegetables such as carrots, peppers, and celery. You can even get some of your veggies in peanut butter, almond butter, or hummus.
- a low carb fruit and a half of a protein bar.
- one cup of cottage cheese, six almonds, and one-quarter cup of blueberries or strawberries.
- grilled chicken breast left over from your barbecue the night before (Drizzle on a little olive oil and add a little salt and pepper—very yummy.)
- a bottle of water and perhaps a cup of green tea. (Sweeten your tea with Splenda or Stevia.)
- a few slices of lean turkey rolled up and dipped into salsa or Dijon mustard.
- a small lettuce salad with cottage cheese, five small almonds, and a tablespoon of oil with balsamic vinegar.

Many people get a sweet tooth late at night, and it is important to avoid sweets before bedtime. Elevated blood sugars just before bedtime will make sleeping difficult.

SURVIVAL GUIDE FOR WEEKENDS, RESTAURANTS, AND OTHER GASTRONOMIC ADVENTURES

It is difficult, at best, to implement a radical change in eating patterns and habits that have developed over years. They are re-inforced through interactions with family, friends, and society. Life presents us with several opportunities to fall off the food wagon. Temptation and cravings can be intense, and it pays to have a few tricks up your sleeve to rescue you, especially early on. Here are a few tips that will help to make your transition to a healthy lifestyle less painful:

JUST SAY "NO" TO CHIPS

When you are at your favorite Mexican restaurant and the waiter walks out with a basket of chips and yummy salsa, just say, "No, thank you." Never let them touch the table. If they are sitting right in front of you, staring at you, *singing* to you, your determination is more likely to fold. That applies to breadbaskets as well. Just say no!

SPLIT THE ENTRÉE

In this world of "Supersize me, please," most restaurants are serving larger and larger portions to satisfy our runaway food addictions. Larger portions mean higher revenues for the food business. When Europeans visit our country, they are amazed at our portion sizes. To cut down on your portion size and save a little money, try splitting the entrée with your companion. You will be surprised at how much less you eat while still being satisfied.

MAKE THE KITCHEN EARN THEIR KEEP

Chefs at high-quality restaurants are happy to modify the menu for you. Request that they use oil in place of butter. Ask them to leave off creamy or cheesy sauces. Ask for sauces on the side, instead.

DON'T GET SIDETRACKED

Don't get carried away with side orders. Choose plain grilled vegetables such as asparagus, beans, etc. Request that your vegetables be steamed, rather soaked in a puddle of butter. Request a plain sweet potato instead of the sugary marshmallow-covered variety. Mashed potatoes or any other potato variant is a no-no. (Did you know that a French fry is a potato?)

DITCH ALL FRIED FOODS

No exceptions to this rule. Nothing good comes from fried foods. Super-heated frying oils are outright poisons. They are nothing more than health bombs. Avoid them like the plague.

EAT LIMITED AMOUNTS OF LEAN RED MEAT

Large amounts of cholesterol-laden high-fat meats are not friendly to your cardiovascular system. Try to limit red meat to once or twice a week. When you eat meat, choose a lean variety of no more than eight ounces, preferably six ounces. Never consume the fatty, marbled cuts that are full of artery-clogging fats and cholesterol. This means that prime rib, cheeseburgers, hot dogs, and deli meats have to go!

CHEAT DAY

Most mere mortals shudder at the thought of living the rest of their lives devoid of life's little culinary pleasures. Treat yourself to a cheat day once every ten to twelve days to keep your brain from rebelling. You can do almost anything consistently for ten to twelve days. Another way, as suggested by Dr. Loren Corain, founder of the Paleo diet, is to eat clean 85 percent of the time. That gives you 15 percent for dietary "sin." I recommend you sin big; get it out of your system. A regular sabbatical from a disciplined dietary plan will keep you from feeling deprived with little overall effect on your long-term health goals. The important thing is to get right back on track. The key to success in eating your way to a long, healthy life free from chronic disease is to design a healthy nutritional plan and stick to it. Cheat days are a nice little reward for hanging in there and doing the right thing.

OTHER ASSORTED LAST-MINUTE THOUGHTS

- Stop buying foods labeled low fat. Low fat usually *always* means higher carbohydrates.
- Never eat a carbohydrate by itself. Always combine it with a protein and preferably some fiber to slow its release into the bloodstream.
- Stop drinking your calories. Sodas, alcohol, and fruit juices are all high in sugar and go straight into your bloodstream. Diet sodas are no better; in many ways, they're worse.
- Always be asking yourself this burning question: "What is this thing I'm about to eat going to do my blood sugar?" Remember that elevated blood sugar is the genesis of a chain reaction of events that leads to a whole score of chronic diseases that are largely preventable. Your body craves it—but it is bad medicine. Protect yourself from *yourself*! Exercise your gift of choice!
- Fats are not the devil. They are a vital component to your diet. They are essential to your cells and help with activating a sense of satiety. Remember that dietary fat plays essentially no role in obesity. The best sources of fat are from fish, seeds, and nuts. Bad fats are to be avoided. Learn what they are. Always avoid trans fats and hydrogenated oils found in fried or baked foods. Finally, fats are a very concentrated source of calories, so be careful how much you eat.

PUTTING IT ALL TOGETHER

Follow a Mediterranean diet. Eat small snacks at midmorning, midafternoon, and midevening to feed your metabolic engine and keep it hot. Think of food as a tool to control your metabolic engine and influence your hormones and other systems to your advantage. Oh, and did I mention—*avoid carbs*?

Remember that well-balanced nutrition is the most important factor in your overall health—in fact, it's critical to your success. The foods you consume on a daily basis are powerful drugs. The right choices profoundly influence your health and quality of life. Poor nutritional choices will doom you to failure, regardless of how much you exercise, how balanced your hormones are, or how many supplements you take. Understand this and you will be successful!

CHAPTER 8

SUPPLEMENTS: SNAKE OIL OR SCIENCE?

*D*o you take vitamins? How many do you take and what kind? Are they taxing your liver, or helping you to maintain health?

Vitamins consist of a group of thirteen organic compounds. Vitamins are very important because they ensure normal growth and development. They play a significant part in our overall health acting as hormone messengers, regulating tissue growth, and cell differentiation, and serving as antioxidants. They are responsible for the function of many of our critical chemical reactions. We can't make them in any sufficient quantity ourselves. Many of us do not eat foods that contain enough of them, or we eat foods that are lacking them altogether.

There are those, however, who believe that vitamins and supplements are not necessary. They feel if you eat a "healthy and wholesome diet," you're getting all you need. Some go way out on a limb and claim they are harmful to us—that they even create disease and can cause death.

Every now and then, you see a "scientific study" that warns us about the dangerous effects of various supplements. Many of these reports ignored why patients started taking supplements in the first place! Some included patients who were in poor health and started taking supplements but already had an increased risk of illness and death from all causes, regardless of whether or not they took supplements. Many of the studies looked at a very specific, skewed population, making it impossible to render valid conclusions for the population as a whole. Frequently, the quality, quantity, or form of the vitamins used in the studies was not standard or what is used in real-life practice.

We all can agree that unsupervised and uninformed use of vitamins can carry some risk. However, it is clear from years of quality research that the benefits of supplements far outweigh the risks. At a time when thousands lose their lives every day from taking properly prescribed medications from their doctors, supplements are relatively safe.

VITAMIN HISTORY WE LEARNED IN SCHOOL

In medical school, we learned that recommended levels of nutrients were the minimum levels needed to prevent diseases such as scurvy, rickets, beriberi, or pellagra. Most of these guidelines were established in the 1940s, when our food and soil were very different. They were also established with disease prevention in mind and have little to do with optimum health. For optimum health, mere adherence to the traditional recommended daily allowance (RDA) is grossly inadequate. The sad truth is that many of us have one or more nutrient deficiencies despite consuming sufficient amounts recommended by these obsolete guidelines.

YOUR INDIVIDUAL NEEDS ARE UNIQUE

The nutrients our bodies need vary for each individual. It is truly impossible for the RDA's estimate to meet the needs of everyone. Supplements, therefore, are needed to replenish specific nutritional deficiencies. Some may need more than others.

Your unique needs, specific activities, environmental exposure, specific stressful or emotional times in life, and health conditions may result in higher needs for certain nutrients. For example, protein and carb needs are greater for athletic competition; folic acid needs tend to be higher during pregnancy, while menopausal women may be vulnerable to calcium deficiencies.

A body suffering from inflammation, which occurs in cases of all chronic pain or disease, requires more of many nutrients than a healthy body. Your activities, age, sex, and health conditions are uniquely your own, so your needs are not the same and will vary over time.

WHY DO WE NEED SUPPLEMENTS?

We evolved from eating wild foods containing dramatically higher levels of all vitamins, minerals, and essential fats. Because of depleted soils, industrial farming, and crop hybridization, the animals and vegetables we eat have fewer nutrients. Processed factory-made foods, though convenient and tasty, have almost no nutrients. The modern burden of environmental toxins and lifestyle factors such as lack of sunlight and chronic stress lead to higher nutrient needs.

The US Department of Health and Human Services has shown that the typical American diet does not always provide a sufficient level of vitamins and minerals. In today's culture, most of us eat processed, easy-to-grab foods that are high in calories and low in nutrition. We tend to eat based on what we prefer, and our preference is often based on flavor and convenience, rather than nutrient richness. Subsequently, we all have deficiencies, and therefore, potential illness. We eat low nutrient, high calorie foods that are highly processed, hybridized, genetically altered, shipped long distances, and grown in nutrient-depleted soil.

As a matter of fact, large-scale nutritional deficiencies in our population, including omega-3 fats, vitamin D, folate, zinc, magnesium, and iron, have been well documented in government-sponsored research projects. Supplements are not a replacement for food, but they can give the less-than-stellar diet that extra edge. And they work.

A CLOSER LOOK AT WHY EVERYONE NEEDS SUPPLEMENTS TO STAY HEALTHY

Environmental Toxins

We live in a soup of toxins; they are inescapable. The US Environmental Protection Agency published in 2002 that more than 7.1 billion pounds of 650 different chemicals had been released into the air or water. Researchers found that the blood of the subjects contained nearly one hundred chemicals that did not exist forty years ago.

At birth, babies born in the US have an average of 200 foreign chemicals in their bodies.

Toxic exposure happens throughout your day (sunscreen; fragrances; cosmetics; hair color; smog; cleaning products; outgassing from new carpets, paints, plastics, and construction materials; pesticides; etc.) and requires specific nutrients to enable you to process its effects. These nutrients are used to help the liver detoxify; they then combine with the toxins to help eliminate them from the system.

FARMING PRACTICES THAT TRASH YOUR FOOD

Soil Depletion

In the post-World War II era, commercial farmers began replacing standard mulch and manure fertilizers with nitrogen (N), phosphorus (P), and potassium (K) fertilizer. Over time, the NPK fertilizer yielded crops that were deficient in many essential micronutrients. Studies reveal that the nutritional values in food have declined significantly over the past seventy-five years. Since 1950, levels of calcium, riboflavin, vitamin C, iron, potassium, and protein in vegetables and fruits have declined significantly.

Hybrid Crops

Hybrid crops yield more food per acre. At least ten times as much rice or wheat are grown on the same land as one hundred years ago, but the land is not stocked with ten times the minerals, vitamins, and other nutrients. As a result, today's wheat contains about 6 percent protein, whereas one hundred years ago, it contained 12 to 14 percent. Trace mineral levels are similarly much lower due to high-yield farming methods.

Chemical Pesticides and Herbicides

Chemical pesticides and herbicides make food toxic and damage soil microorganisms. Soil microorganisms are needed to make minerals and other nutrients available to plants. So the plant becomes deficient. Our bodies also require extra nutrients to process pesticide residues that remain inside the foods. Some of these agents contain lead, arsenic, and other toxic metals that slowly accumulate in the body.

LONG DISTANCE TRANSPORTATION OF FOOD DIMINISHES NUTRITIONAL CONTENT

As soon as a food is harvested, the levels of certain nutrients begin to diminish. Today, many foods are grown thousands of miles from population centers. They are shipped long distances and are stored for long periods of time, causing depletion of important B-complex and C vitamins.

NUTRITIONAL DEPLETION IN FOOD PREPARATION

Food processing often drastically reduces the nutrient content of common foods such as wheat flour, rice, dairy products, and others. For example, the refining of wheat to make white flour removes 80 percent of its magnesium, 70 to 80 percent of its zinc, 87 percent of its chromium, 88 percent of its manganese, and 50 percent of its cobalt.

Similarly, refining sugarcane to make white sugar removes 99 percent of its magnesium and 93 percent of its chromium. Polishing (refining) rice removes 75 percent of its zinc and chromium.

Pasteurization and homogenization of dairy products drastically reduces the bioavailability of calcium, phosphorus, and some proteins in milk and other dairy products.

FOOD ADDITIVES

Thousands of artificial flavors; colors; sweeteners; artificial sweeteners; stabilizers; flavor enhancers, like MSG; emulsifiers; hardeners; softeners; chemical preservatives; and other chemicals are added to most people's food today. Many are toxic, and many diminish the nutritional content of the food.

POOR DIGESTION

If our digestive systems functioned optimally, we wouldn't

need as many high-quality nutrients in supplement form—but that is not the case. It is estimated that one half of the US population produces insufficient stomach acid, which diminishes the ability to absorb nutrients from food and can increase inflammation, stomach bacteria, and numerous other health issues such as bloating, stomach pain, and even depression.

Today almost everyone's digestion is very weak. This is due to eating poor quality food, hybridized varieties of foods like wheat, and having to digest and handle so many refined foods and chemicals in the foods. It is also due to low vitality, low digestive enzyme secretion, imbalanced intestinal flora, and intestinal infections like yeast that are extremely common.

As a result, most people do not absorb nutrients well at all. This further impairs nutrient levels in the body and increases nutritional needs.

STRESSFUL LIFESTYLES

Our overwhelmingly busy lifestyles impair digestion and use up more nutrients. These may include calcium, magnesium, zinc, chromium, and manganese deficiencies, among others. Zinc, for example, begins to be eliminated from the body within minutes of a stressful event.

PHARMACEUTICALS AND OVER-THE-COUNTER DRUGS

Drugs like Ibuprofen and antacids knock both our acid and base balance out of whack. This reduces the breakdown of food and decreases absorption of nutrients. They can also break down our intestinal lining, leading to malabsorption and food sensitivities. Antibiotics knock out "good" bacteria essential for digestion. When digestion is compromised, fewer nutrients are utilized.

THE BOTTOM LINE

Ultimately, the question is not how much of a certain nutrient or vitamin you need to avoid illness, but how much you need to be optimally healthy! The current vitamin recommendations are not accurate. They are based on disease prevention, rather than optimal health. They can no longer be said to be biologically relevant!

In today's world, **everyone** needs a basic multivitamin and mineral supplement. The research is overwhelming on this point. In fact, thousands of patients have nutrient deficiencies.

I have found that by correcting these deficiencies, people feel better, are in a better mood, are sharper mentally, and have better memory and focus. Patients treated for deficiencies have more energy, resolve chronic health complaints or conditions, and even lose weight. Taking supplements also helps prevent disease.

The basic vitamin recommendations outlined below include nutrients that form the backbone for proper optimal biological function, robust health, and healthy aging. These nutrients work as a team. The basic workhorse team outlined below should be taken by everyone.

SUPPLEMENTS YOU SHOULD TAKE EVERY DAY

THIS REALLY IS THE BOTTOM LINE!!

Here are the supplements I recommend for everyone, every day:

1. A high-quality multivitamin.
2. Calcium-magnesium, with at least 600 mg of calcium and 400 mg of magnesium. The calcium should be calcium citrate or chelated versions of minerals. Do not use calcium carbonate or magnesium oxide, which are cheap minerals that are poorly absorbed.

3. Vitamin D3: 5,000 IU a day (people who are deficient in vitamin D will need more).

4. Omega-3 fatty acids that contain the fats EPA and DHA: 2,000 to 4,000 mg a day.

5. CoQ10: 100 mg a day. This feeds your mitochondria (your cells' energy factories).

6. Resveratrol, which is a strong antioxidant to help reverse the *rusting* of your body due to aging effects of everyday metabolism. Recommended dosage is 100 to 200 mg per day.

7. A high-quality probiotic. This will keep the bugs in your gut friendly.

The cost is low, the benefit is high, and the risk is non-existent for these nutritional supplements. Not only will you feel better, have better immune function, and improve your energy and brain function, you will also prevent many problems on down the road. **So eat a healthy diet—and take your nutritional supplements every day. It is essential for lifelong, vibrant health.**

BE A SAVVY SHOPPER

The most expensive supplement on the market is the one that doesn't work!! Supplements are a multi-billion dollar unregulated industry. The wide display of choices in drugstores, food stores, online, and even in doctors' offices can make your head spin! It is now more important than ever to be aware of what you are and are not getting.

Be sure to pick quality supplements—ones that contain nutrients and compounds research has shown to be effective and safe. Think of them as part of your diet. You want the best quality food and supplements you can buy.

Because I use supplements in my practice as a cornerstone

of healing and repair, I have investigated supplement makers, toured their factories, studied independent analysis of their finished products, and experimented with them personally.

I have learned there are few companies I can rely on. I want my patients to heal and get their life back, so I need to be very cautious when evaluating what I recommend

This is how I judge quality supplements:

1. The form of the nutrient is high in quality, is well absorbed, or used by the body.
2. The dosage on the label matches the dose in the pill.
3. They contain absolutely no additives, colors, fillers, and allergens.
4. The raw materials (especially herbs) have been tested for toxins like mercury or lead and are consistently pure from batch to batch.
5. The factory in which they are produced follows good manufacturing standards, so products are uniformly consistent in quality. I want to be sure I know I'm getting the same thing every time.

In my experience, Designs for Health and Metagenics are the industry leaders and the gold standard by which all other supplement manufacturers should be compared.

DETAILS OF MY FAVORITE SUPPLEMENTS

Coenzyme Q10 (CoQ10) is an essential component of healthy mitochondrial function. It is incorporated into the cells' mitochondria throughout the body where it facilitates and regulates the oxidation of fats and sugars into energy. Aging adults have been found to have over 50 percent less CoQ10 on average, compared to that of young adults. This finding makes CoQ10 one of the most important nutrients for people over 30 to supplement with. About 95 percent of cellular energy is produced in the mitochondria. The mitochondria are the cells' "energy powerhouses," and many maladies have been referred to as "mitochondrial disorders." A growing body of scientific research links a deficiency of CoQ10 to age-related mitochondrial disorders.

This is a wonderful product to enhance energy levels in anyone between 50 and 60 years of age. It is also excellent for cardiac patients, in particular, and may have other uses as well. Definitely take it if you insist on taking a "statin" drug because this class of drugs depletes CoQ10, which is very dangerous. I never recommend these drugs, by the way. Natural alternatives are far better and just as effective in most cases (such as red rice yeast or chromium or more fiber).

Fish Oil can reduce deaths from heart disease. Studies on omega-3 fatty acids are so impressive that an agency of the National Institutes of Health published a report stating this fact. The FDA itself states supportive (but not conclusive) research shows that consumption of EPA and DHA omega-3 fatty acids may actually reduce the risk of coronary heart disease.

There are several mechanisms attributed to fish oil's beneficial effects. The latest government report cites the triglyceride-lowering effects of fish oil on reducing heart and blood vessel disorders. Another beneficial mechanism of fish oil is to protect healthy blood flow in arteries. In addition, it is good for skin and hair, the heart, cholesterol, neurologic states such as depression, ADD, ADHD and most other neurological disorders.

Probiotics are friendly bacteria that have a positive influence on the immune system (60% of our immune system resides within the gut), digestive system, vitamin production, and detoxification. Destroyers of good bacteria are antibiotics, chlorinated water, antacids, high sugar diets, and diets high in refined and processed foods.

Multivitamins are important for everyone to take. Industrial food processing depletes soil of nutrients, and food processing destroys vitamins A, B, D, E, and many minerals. Seventy-four percent of Americans do not eat the recommended eight servings of fruits and vegetables daily.

Vitamin D deficiency is now epidemic in the United States. At risk groups for vitamin D deficiency are dark skinned individuals, hospitalized patients, those who are obese, and the elderly. Vitamin D tunes up the immune system helping with cancer surveillance and has also have been shown to hinder cancer growth.

Calcium and Magnesium are minerals that are both good for bones, hair, nails, heart, thyroid, and leg cramps. Magnesium is needed by most people due to dietary deficiencies. We give it with calcium to everyone. Extra magnesium may be used, at times, based on a high calcium/magnesium ratio, faster oxidation rate, to help with difficult cases of constipation, and perhaps for leg cramps and some cardiovascular conditions. .

Magnesium is safe in tablet form. The dosage orally is 250 to 1,000 mg daily. Too much will cause diarrhea.

Antioxidants play an important role in the destruction of free radicals. They also reduce oxidative stress in the body and slow the aging process.

CHAPTER 9

EXERCISE: THE ONE-HOUR PLAN TO FIT AND HEALTHY

WHAT'S YOUR EXERCISE PROGRAM LOOK LIKE?

The word "exercise" conjures up images of ellipticals, treadmills. and other pieces of dreary equipment that are meant to aid you in your exercise routine. The good news is that they are not the only means to better physical fitness. Carrying out an activity that is meant to improve your physical well-being is the essence of exercising, and it could mean anything from using the stairs instead of the elevator, or walking to your local store instead of taking the car, or taking part in a physically challenging event like a triathlon.

Exercise has numerous benefits, and recent research has found that people differ depending upon their expectations of exercise. Cornelius and colleagues, in a study published in the *Journal of Health Psychology*, found that some people were motivated by health benefits of exercise, while others were solely motivated by the appearance aspect of exercise. So if your wife agrees to go jogging with you every morning, she may not just be concerned about getting your system into shape, but is hoping to look more fit herself!

There is no doubt that regular exercise enhances physical appearance: double chins give way to smart jaws and love handles melt away to a more graceful figure. If this catches your eye, then we know which side of the bandwagon you're on.

In our modern digital world, we have definitely seen a decrease in our activity levels—especially as we age. There are too many neat timesaving tools that make activity unnecessary. A huge decrease in activity is common starting around age 45. Only 35 percent of people aged 45 or older engage in regular physical activity. The reasons for this could fill a book, but time constraints, family and job commitments, progressive fatigue, and chronic stress all contribute to our tendency to put exercise on the back burner.

Yet years of research and thousands of studies on human populations in health and longevity all confirm this fact: *exercise is medicine.* The common thread seen in all cultures demonstrating impressive health and longevity statistics is that they remain active throughout their entire lives. Research has proven that there is a strong likelihood of fair to poor health tomorrow if we live a sedentary lifestyle today.

REASONS PEOPLE DON'T EXERCISE

Urbanization has significantly altered people's behavior patterns. As more of the population moves to cities, population overcrowding, high-density traffic, and lack of parks lead to a less active lifestyle. I know that in Dallas, Texas, where I live, an hour-long commute in rush-hour traffic each way is not unusual. And every good soccer mom or dad would have to hide in shame if they didn't constantly taxi their children to multiple afterschool events to optimally expand their child's horizons. Behavioral changes, such as driving our children to school, have become increasingly popular (I mean, kids don't even walk a mile these days). Work cycles have become more demanding and many people take their work home leaving them less and less free time. The bottom line is that people have less time during the day, and they are beat when they get home.

Increase in use of electronics has led to a decrease of physical activity. Worldwide, with the introduction of the Information Age and the passing of the Industrial Age, there has been a large shift towards less physically demanding work. This has been accompanied by increasing use of mechanized transportation, a greater prevalence of labor-saving technology in the home, and recreational pursuits that are less physical. The sheer number of available "digital distraction" entertainment in the home is mind numbing. Tearing my kids away from a marathon session of *Call to Duty* or *Halo* is virtually impossible. I have friends who can recite the ESPN sports TV schedule by heart.

WHY YOU WANT TO EXERCISE

Exercise is extremely important in preventing declines in our health. As you look around you at our society, you can clearly see what happens when we abandon exercise as part of our daily routine. Chronic degenerative disease and obesity is rampant, but it doesn't have to be. Regular exercise can help protect you from:
- heart disease and stroke
- high blood pressure
- diabetes
- obesity
- osteoporosis

- back pain
- insomnia
- mood disorders and depression
- stress

THE SPECIFICS: A SYSTEMS VIEW

THE CARDIOVASCULAR SYSTEM

The beneficial effect of exercise on the cardiovascular system is well documented. There is a direct correlation between physical inactivity and cardiovascular mortality, and physical inactivity is an independent risk factor for the development of coronary artery disease. People who remain sedentary have the highest risk for all-cause and cardiovascular disease mortality.

HEART DISEASE AND STROKE

Daily physical activity can help prevent heart disease and stroke by strengthening your heart muscle, lowering your blood pressure, raising your high-density lipoprotein (HDL) levels (good cholesterol), and lowering low-density lipoprotein (LDL) levels (bad cholesterol), thereby improving blood flow.

In a study published in the *Journal of Adolescent Health* in its February 2014 issue, researchers Dulfer and colleagues analyzed study participants aged between 10 and 25 years born with heart defects (congenital malformations). Some of the study participants were allowed to take up a controlled exercise program, while the others formed the control group. This study found that study participants who undertook the exercise program displayed better cognitive ability and improved social functioning. So even if you have a congenital heart malformation, there is no excuse to avoid a well-monitored exercise regime.

HIGH BLOOD PRESSURE

If raging blood pressure has been preventing you from taking up exercise, you may be interested to learn that regular physical activity can actually reduce blood pressure. Blood pressure was significantly reduced after six months of exercise in obese individuals, as detailed in a study conducted by Farah and colleagues and published in the *Journal of Pediatric Obesity* in its February 2013 issue.

OBESITY

Physical activity helps to reduce body fat by building or preserving muscle mass and improving the body's ability to use calories. When physical activity is combined with proper nutrition, it can help control weight and prevent obesity, a major risk factor for many diseases.

OSTEOPOROSIS

Women are at a high risk for osteoporosis, especially after menopause. This condition is characterized by a lot of movement restrictions due to pain and frequent fractures as the bones become brittle. Exercise benefits women with osteoporosis as it reduces body weight, which in turn places less stress on the joints and bones. Paolucci and colleagues carried out a study to determine if exercise helps reduce pain in women with osteoporosis; this study was published in the journal *Ageing Clinical and Experimental Research*. The study, which was conducted on sixty women, found that monitored exercise programs helped reduce back pain and improved functional ability of women with osteoporosis, which resulted in a better quality of life.

PSYCHOLOGICAL EFFECTS

Regular physical activity can improve your mood and the

way you feel about yourself. Researchers also have found that exercise is likely to reduce depression and anxiety and help you better manage stress.

IMMUNE SYSTEM

Epidemiological evidence suggests that moderate exercise has a beneficial effect on the immune system. Biomarkers of inflammation (such as C-reactive protein) which are associated with chronic diseases are reduced in active individuals relative to sedentary individuals, and the positive effects of exercise may be due to its anti-inflammatory effects.

BRAIN FUNCTION

A 2008 review of cognitive enrichment therapies (strategies to slow or reverse cognitive decline) concluded that "physical activity, and aerobic exercise in particular, enhances older adults' cognitive function."

In addition, physical activity has been shown to be neuroprotective in many neurodegenerative and neuromuscular diseases, reducing the risk for dementia.

DEPRESSION

When a person exercises, their levels of circulating serotonin and endorphins both increase. These levels are known to stay elevated even several days after exercise is discontinued, possibly contributing to improvement in mood, increased self-esteem, and weight management. Exercise alone is a potential prevention method and/or treatment for mild forms of depression.

The depressed adolescents treated with exercise (DATE) study conducted by H. W. Hughes and colleagues and published in the journal *Ageing Clinical and Experimental Research* devised a standardized aerobic exercise to treat depression in adolescents. The results of this study proved conclusively that exercise improved depression in adolescents and helped them at school as well as in social settings.

SLEEP

A 2010 review of published scientific research suggested that exercise generally improves sleep for most people and helps sleep disorders such as insomnia. The optimum time to exercise may be four to eight hours before bedtime, though exercise at any time of day is beneficial, with the possible exception of heavy exercise right before bedtime, which may disturb sleep.

A study published in the journal *Physiology and Behavior* in the August 2013 issue by researcher C. W. Lang and colleagues explored the influence of exercise on sleep. It was found that physical activity not only promoted sleep, but it improved the quality of sleep by reducing insomnia and wakening at night. So in order to sleep better, exercise better.

Exercise has numerous health benefits as evidenced, and almost every aspect of health is improved as a result of regular exercise. Neuro-degenerative illnesses (like Alzheimer's and Parkinson's) which threaten to disrupt quality of life are delayed to a large extent by exercising regularly. Not only are diseases and illnesses delayed, but the hormones like oxytocin that are secreted after a round of exercise can lift your spirits high. There is an almost immediate mood elevation, which is just great. Good health, a great looking body, and a happy disposition: why then do people stay away from exercise? Let's find out.

DEALING WITH COMMON EXERCISE AVOIDANCE EXCUSES

Although we intuitively know that exercise is good for us, we can think of a million reasons to weasel out of it. The funny thing is, we actually convince ourselves that our excuses are valid. Psychologists call this rationalization and denial. So here are some ideas to help turn your justifications into action!

EXERCISE EXCUSE NO. 1: "I DON'T HAVE TIME."

Really? How much time do you spend surfing the Internet on your computer? How much TV do you watch?. Hit the off switch, and gift yourself an extra thirty to sixty minutes a day to take care of yourself. If you're working long hours, try exercising on the job. Close your office door and jump rope for ten minutes, or walk in place. Get up a half hour earlier, and walk around the block a couple times. Can't get to a gym? Try making small lifestyle changes that help you move more: take the stairs instead of the escalator, don't drive when you can walk, and get a pedometer and try to increase the number of steps you take throughout the day. Make a daily appointment with yourself that is sacred and unbreakable—even if it's only for ten minutes. When you feel you don't have time to spare is when you really need to find the time for *yourself.*

EXCUSE NO. 2: "I'M TOO TIRED."

It may sound counterintuitive, but working out actually gives you more energy. It may help to work out in the morning, before you get wiped out by a demanding workday. But if you're just not a morning person, just do it whenever you feel best. Once you get moving, your fatigue may likely disappear. Try not to exercise too close to bedtime, as exercise could have you all charged up and in no mood for sleep.

EXERCISE EXCUSE NO. 3: "I DON'T GET A BREAK FROM THE KIDS."

Take the kids with you. While they're playing, you can walk

around the playground or jump rope. Walk the kids to school instead of driving them. During their soccer games or practices, walk briskly or jog around the field. Not only is this a great way to bond with your kids, but you are also teaching them the right thing at the right age—to get out and play.

EXERCISE EXCUSE NO. 4: "EXERCISE IS BORING."

Find an activity you enjoy. Think outside the box: try in-line skating, dancing, or gardening. Or, if you love music, try ballroom dancing. There is an exercise for everyone—it can be very enjoyable and doesn't have to be a drag. Find a partner to work with you, or join a group activity. That way, if you slack off, there are others to keep your motivation levels high.

EXERCISE EXCUSE NO. 5: "I JUST DON'T LIKE TO MOVE."

If exercise is painful, try starting by exercising in water. The stronger you get, the easier it will be to support your own body weight, and the less you'll hurt. If you don't like to move because you feel too fat, start with an activity that's less public, like using an exercise video at home. Walk with nonjudgmental friends in your neighborhood while wearing clothes that provide enough coverage that you feel comfortable. In time, as you begin to enjoy what you do, you will learn to be happy with yourself and how you look.

EXERCISE EXCUSE NO. 6: "I ALWAYS END UP QUITTING."

Set small, attainable goals. Then you're more likely to feel like a success, not a failure. If you exercise for five minutes a day for a week, you'll feel good—and more likely to want to try ten minutes a day the next week. It also helps to keep a log and post it somewhere public. Having an exercise buddy keeps you accountable as well, When you back out of a scheduled workout, you're letting down your buddy as well as yourself.

And look toward the future. It's actually harder to start exercising than it is to stick with it once you have your momentum going,

GETTING STARTED

First and foremost, recognize this: one size doesn't fit all. And doing something is *always* better than doing nothing. Everywhere you look, you'll find advice from experts and amateurs alike on how to get and stay fit. Lots of this advice is conflicting. There are as many opinions on how to get and stay fit and how to exercise as there are trainers. Most of the controversy focuses on the minutia of training and is not really material to the overall theme of what you are trying to accomplish. Don't let this confuse or intimidate you; the important thing is to start a plan that works for you. That is how we can get and keep you healthy well into your 70s and 80s. And remember: it's important to get clearance from your physician prior to starting an exercise program.

Don't look for inspiration from movie stars or models; most of them have their photographs airbrushed or photo shopped, and they don't look like that in person most of the time. If you do want a role model, start with a friend or a colleague who has successfully worked at getting fit. They will help you with useful tips and ways to stay on track.

Read as much as you can about fitness. A study conducted by Pankratow and colleagues and published in *PLos One* states just that: it examined the impact of exercise articles. The results? People are actively motivated to exercise after reading a good health or fitness article.

So push everything away, and set aside some time for yourself. Breaking the process into the following four steps will help you ease into the world of fitness . . . where a fitter and healthier body is in store.

Step One: Set aside time each day to exercise. Remember: getting started can often be the most difficult part of any exercise routine. Scheduling exercise into your day and making it a priority will increase the chance of it being successful. If you need to, start small and commit to only ten minutes a day. The idea is to keep a regular routine. Expand the amount of time spent exercising based on your comfort level and availability.

Step Two: Choose activities that you enjoy, such as swimming, biking, or playing tennis or racquetball with friends. Physical activity can be accumulated through a variety of activities.

Step Three: Start with ten to fifteen minutes of exercise activity daily. Each week, add five minutes to your exercise routine until you reach thirty minutes of moderate intensity for a minimum of five days per week.

Step Four: Incorporate strength training into your routine. Sometimes it's a good idea to meet with a physical trainer who can show you the ropes about how to use weights and other resistance devices properly.

There are different types of exercises, and staying with a regimen is dependent on how comfortable you are with a particular form of exercise. Try out various forms of exercise, and find the one that best suit your needs.

TYPES OF EXERCISE

Physical exercise can generally be grouped into three types:

Aerobic exercises focus on increasing cardiovascular endurance and include activities such as running, cycling, walking, swimming, rowing, jumping rope, hiking, or playing tennis.

Anaerobic exercises increase muscle strength and include activities such as weight training and high-intensity interval training.

Flexibility exercises, such as stretching, improve the range of motion of your joints and muscles.

AEROBIC FITNESS

Aerobic refers to the use of oxygen to meet the energy demands of exercise using aerobic metabolism. These are generally light to moderate intensity activities that can be performed over extended periods of time. For example, running a long distance at a moderate pace is an aerobic exercise, but sprinting is not. It is most common for aerobic exercises to involve the leg muscles, primarily or exclusively. Aerobic exercise primarily burns fat. The benefits of regular aerobic exercise are:

- strengthening the muscles of respiration
- strengthening the heart and improving its efficiency
- improving circulation and reducing blood pressure
- improving mental health by reducing stress
- burning body fat and building and strengthening muscle

A GOOD AEROBIC PLAN

If you have been inactive for a while, you may want to start with less strenuous activities such as walking or swimming at a comfortable pace. Beginning at a slow pace, even if it's only for ten minutes a day, will allow you to get into a routine and advance without straining your body. Once you are in better shape, you can step it up.

The experts recommend that you do thirty to sixty minutes of moderate aerobic activity three or four times a week. You want to achieve a target heart rate of 50 to 70 percent of your maximum heart rate (MHR). OK, what's MHR? Start with the number 220 and subtract your age. THAT number is your maximum heart rate (MHR). Now multiply that number by .5 or .7 to get your target heart rate for moderate aerobic activity. For a 50-year-old, MHR = 220 – 50 = 170. So the target heart rate for exercise will be 170 X .7 = 119. There are lots of cheap heart rate monitors you can buy to help you calculate this.

Alternatively, you can do twenty minutes of vigorous aerobic activity three days a week. The target heart rate for this type of activity is 70 to 85 percent of your MHR.

ANAEROBIC TRAINING

HIGH INTENSITY INTERVAL TRAINING (HIIT)

One thing that has become evident is the trend to drift away from the traditional recommendations of long, slow cardio training. High intensity interval training (HIIT) has much greater endurance and calorie-burning benefits and creates less wear and tear on your body. HIIT is a form of cardiovascular exercise. It maximizes both aerobic and anaerobic fitness, while standard cardio training only addresses aerobic fitness.

The sessions can vary from nine to twenty minutes and are very intense. They consist of a warm-up period, followed by six to ten repetitions of very high intensity exercise (near maximum intensity), separated by medium intensity (50 percent) exercise, and ending with a cool-down period. This is an excellent way to maximize a workout on limited time.

HIT maximizes the amount of calories you burn during your exercise session and afterward because it increases the length of time it takes your body to recover from each exercise session. Your body continues to burn calories for up to forty-eight hours after you work out.

RESISTANCE TRAINING

These exercises cause muscles to contract against an external resistance. The goal is to gradually and progressively overload the musculoskeletal system so that it gets stronger. Resistance training works by causing microscopic damage or tears to the muscle cells, which are quickly repaired by the body to help the muscles regenerate and grow stronger. Resistance training is primarily an anaerobic activity. Besides increasing muscle strength and muscle mass, resistance training increases and maintains bone density, increases your metabolic rate, and raises your hormonal response. Remember that your muscles heal and grow when you are working out, so it's important to build in time between workouts for recovery.

WHY DO RESISTANCE TRAINING?

The benefits of resistance training are well documented. In ancient societies, humans got a workout by building shelters, hunting, farming, and in undertaking all the other activities of daily life. Today, however, we have engineered inactivity into our lives with labor saving devices to the extent that our muscles rarely need to be pushed very hard. We don't rake leaves or cut grass or shovel snow by hand; we often spend more time in front of our computers and televisions than we do outdoors. Humans lose five pounds of muscle every decade after the age of 30. So we need something to build those muscles and keep them big and strong.

Resistance exercise can slow down or even reverse the aging process by building muscle mass and strength. Resistance training has also been shown to build bone. This is important because in our society, osteoporosis is a big player and can be a crippling disease. Resistance exercise also raises the metabolic rate, which is another important factor in maintaining body weight. The benefits of weight training for older people have been confirmed by studies of people who began engaging in it even in their 80s and 90s. Stronger muscles improve posture, provide better support for joints, and reduce the risk of injury from everyday activities.

RESISTANCE 101

Beginners are often confused as to whether they should use free weights or machines. Others like resistance bands or even use their own body weight. The truth is that all of these methods work great. No one method of resistance exercise is superior. As long as your muscles are contracting against external resistance, the exercises will work to build your strength and tone. Each method has advantages and disadvantages.

FREE WEIGHTS (DUMBBELLS AND BARBELLS)

These allow for less confined movement than machines and allow you to recruit more muscles during exercise. The disadvantage is that there is a risk of injury from dropped bars or dumbbells, and they can be costly to purchase.

MACHINES

Machines are simple to use and relatively safe. They don't require a lot of coordination. They do require a lot of space and are expensive.

EXERCISE TUBING

Exercise tubing consists of elastic tubes with handles. They come in various thicknesses to increase the tension. They are very inexpensive and versatile. They are portable, and you can pack them in your bag for vacation, or leave them in your office and use them during short breaks at work. The only real disadvantage is that they lose some of their elasticity over time.

BODY WEIGHT

Push-ups, sit-ups, chin-ups, squat thrusts, lunges, and step-ups are just some of the exercises you can do using your own body weight. The advantage of these exercises is that you can do them almost anywhere.

DESIGNING A WEIGHT LIFTING PLAN

You need a good program that includes resistance exercises at least two days each week.

Weight: Beginners should start with whatever weight can be lifted eight to twelve times to the point of fatigue while still maintaining good form. Fatigue means that you can't lift the weight one more time with good form.

Sets: Beginners can start with one set per exercise. Advance to three to five sets per exercise as you gain experience.

Time Between Sets: Rest less than one minute between sets if you want to develop endurance and tone. Rest up to three minutes if you want to focus more on strength because extra recovery time allows the muscles to work harder and lift more the next set.

Order of Exercises: You want to exercise your large muscle groups before smaller groups. If you fatigue the smaller groups first, then the larger groups cannot be worked as hard.

Exercises: Select one or two exercises per muscle group. You will eventually want to perform eight to ten exercises per workout covering all major muscle groups.

Rest and Recovery: Allow a day or two between workouts when you first get started so the muscles can recover and grow.

NUTRITION AND RESISTANCE TRAINING

Your diet should be modified to maximize the benefits of resistance training. Adequate protein is required for building skeletal muscle. Water is consumed throughout the course of a workout to prevent dehydration. A protein shake is also consumed during or immediately following the workout because protein uptake and usage are increased at this time. Glucose is often consumed as well since this quickly replenishes glycogen lost during exercise. A good recovery drink should contain glucose, protein (usually whey), and branched-chain amino acids.

FLEXIBILITY TRAINING

Our quality of life is enhanced by improving and maintaining a good range of motion in our joints. Loss of flexibility can be a predisposing factor for issues such as pain syndromes or balance disorders, which can result in injuries. Flexibility activities include:

- **ballistic**: repetitive bouncing movements
- **dynamic**: movements that mimic specific sports or exercise such as high knee lifting, lunges and skipping
- **static**: passively stretching muscle to the point of resistance

Thirty seconds is the minimum time to get the benefits of stretching, whereas two minutes is the maximum. At least thirty minutes of static stretching exercises done twice a week will improve flexibility within five weeks.

Stretching should only be started when your muscles are warmed up and your body temperature is elevated. Increasing this range of motion creates good posture and develops proficient performance of everyday activities that benefit your overall health and longevity.

TIPS FOR SUCCESS

- Be consistent: No exercise program works if you don't do it consistently.
- Set realistic goals.
- Find a buddy: accountability is a great motivator.
- Mix up the workouts to keep yourself from getting bored and to keep your body from adapting.
- Set aside specific dates and times to exercise, and make these appointments sacred.
- Be less concerned with weight loss and what the scale says and more concerned with your percentage of total body fat.
- Keep inspired: fitness is a state of mind.
- Be patient: Rome wasn't built in a day. There will be ups and downs, setbacks and victories. Hang in there, and the rewards will be yours.

One final thing to remember: exercise does not replace nutrition. It's very common to see someone who's working very hard at the gym with a persistent belly pooch. These people think that exercise permits them to pass on a proper diet. That's a big NO. Diet and exercise go hand in hand, and you have to focus on what you put into your body as much as on how you work it.

Eating right is about getting the right amount of nutrition, giving your body the energy to exercise. Slimming down and toning up when you look gaunt and drawn would defeat the whole purpose. Smart, toned abs with a healthy, glowing face is not a dream but a reality—one that you will have to chase down with the right blend of diet and exercise.

Remember: the first step is the only hard part in any fitness regime, and that's getting started. Once the results begin to show, it can become a passion which will drive you to keep striving for more.

CHAPTER 10

SLEEP: THE REDHEADED STEPCHILD OF HEALTH AND WELLNESS

The best cure for insomnia is to get a lot of sleep. —W. C. FIELDS

Ahhh—Sleep! Sleep is something that we all take for granted; that is, until we don't have it. Most of us remember our teenage years, when we would go to bed at two in the morning and sleep until noon the next day. Or, when we were in our early 20s, when a good night's sleep was a welcome reward for a full day of living. Sometimes, we burned our candle bright into the wee hours of the night with little need for sleep. Back then, sleep was for sissies! In our early innocent years, all of us took the luxury of plentiful, restful sleep as a universal given. Then, seemingly out of nowhere, something changed. We noticed that as our days became more demanding, our jobs more stressful, and our family responsibilities more time intensive, those wonderful nights of blissful, restful sleep were more elusive: they became the exception, rather than the rule. For many of us, getting a good night's sleep is a thing of the past. Restful sleep is not just about how many hours you log in the rack, but also about the quality of your zzzzs.

As life gets more complicated, sleep can be an early casualty. In our production-centric, results-oriented, 24/7 overdrive culture, some superstars take boastful pride in the idea that they only need four hours of sleep a night. It somehow makes them feel tough. Others feel they have no choice; they have twenty-eight hours of stuff to accomplish in only twenty-four hours, and something has to give somewhere. In their mind, sleep can be sacrificed because it's a luxury they just can't afford. Still others want to sleep. They go through the motions of going to bed early in eager anticipation of restful slumber. But they find that sleep in elusive. They toss and turn, searching for the magic door to dreamland. Or they fall asleep (frequently with a little pharmaceutical help), only to wake up several times during the night staring at the ceiling, while their minds race through the events of yesterday or the anticipation of tomorrow.

Many of us know that sleep is important, but few understand that quality, restful sleep is **critical**. Sleep deprivation has far-reaching physical and psychological consequences that serve to erode your quality of life and open the door to a gauntlet of degenerative chronic diseases. Lack of adequate sleep is a big player in influencing how effectively you function today and in the prevention of chronic diseases in the future. Solving the sleep problem can often be accomplished through simple lifestyle changes. Others may require the services of a healthcare professional to look under the hood and determine if metabolic imbalances or physical barriers like sleep apnea may be a player in preventing them from sawing logs on a regular basis.

WHAT HAPPENS DURING SLEEP?

What is sleep, anyway? Sleep is a state where you cease being awake (profound, I know) and are in a state of either partial or complete natural suspension of consciousness. Our ancient ancestors believed that sleep was a condition in which the body was half-dead; they believed that none of the organs were actually functioning. However, we now know that it is during sleep that the body's organs and tissues are restored and renewed. It's much like parking the car overnight in a mechanic's garage, only it needs to happen every day. Sleep allows the body to consolidate memories and work on its subconscious mind, which sometimes gives rise to dreams.

Sleep is the time when the body repairs itself. During sleep, you enter an anabolic state. This is the time when you rejuvenate just about everything. The internal organs and nervous and musculoskeletal systems repair nicks and bruises acquired throughout the day, and when growth hormone is secreted, it makes them stronger and more resilient. Critical "restocking" of essential hormones and neurotransmitters takes place. The immune system strengthens and resets. Mental functions, such as memory, cognitive function, learning ability, decision-making, and reasoning ability, reset themselves. New neural connections are formed, making your mental processes more efficient and incorporating what you learned that day. It's all about recharging your biological system (just like a battery), and this will better prepare you to face the next day's challenges.

When sleep is inadequate, your body will be unable to cope, and you will not yet be ready to tackle critical decisions or to concentrate. It will also be difficult to engage or to be actively involved with people around you, resulting in poor self-esteem and lackluster social skills. Is this all a figment of your imagination, or does sleep really play such an important role in your life? A study published in January 2014 in the *Journal of Neuropsychology* states that sleep deprivation affects the behavior, mood, and well-being of even the healthiest of people. This study, performed on sixteen male volunteers, tested their behavior before and after sleep deprivation. It concluded conclusively that sleep deprivation had a negative impact on an individual's behavior and mood.

Everyone knows that poor sleep habits are harmful when you intend to drive; however, recent startling research has revealed that even experienced drivers fare badly after sleep deprivation. In fact, a study published in the journal Traffic Injury Prevention in January 2014 found that professional drivers cope as badly as nonprofessionals after sleep deprivation, indicating that no matter how many miles you have driven or for how many years, when you haven't slept enough, you cannot go the distance! Imagine how this would impact your work performance during an average day at the office.

Sleep also plays a vital role in how well you look; no point in dabbling with assorted night creams when you don't give your skin enough time to renew. When you don't get the right amount of sleep, you tend to look haggard and dull, with dark circles under your eyes (which is great if you are a panda!). A well-rested person tends to look radiant and fresh. So beauty sleep is indeed just that.

WHAT MESSES UP SLEEP?

Among the many causes of sleep deprivation, chronic stress is a biggie. Chronic stress comes in many different packages. Most people can identify with the stress imposed by challenging relationships with family, friends, and coworkers. Financial stress, either because we have trouble paying our bills or from constant demands of the drive for success, can stick in our brains as a relentless companion. For some, worries about yesterday, today, and tomorrow never cease. Environmental stress, from barking dogs, artificial lighting, a noisy environment, toxic chemicals, or something as simple as your spouse keeping the television on till the wee hours of the morning, can be a problem. Concurrent medical conditions such as arthritis, sleep apnea, heart disease, and diabetes place a heavy burden on our limited repair and growth resources and are significant physiologic stressors. These stressors amp up our sympathetic nervous system and place us in a defensive "fight or flight" posture. Our normal peaks and valleys of the stress hormone cortisol are disrupted, our daily rhythms disturbed, and sleep evades us.

Hormone imbalances also are a significant cause of insomnia. Menopause, perimenopause, andropause (male menopause), thyroid imbalances, and adrenal fatigue all manifest themselves by robbing you of a good night's sleep.

Dietary indiscretions, such as raiding the refrigerator for a bowl of ice cream just before bedtime, can spike your blood sugar followed by the 2 a.m. sugar crash, which will wake you up more times than not. Similarly, alcohol consumption just before bed may help put you to sleep initially, but it negatively affects REM sleep and sleep quality will suffer. Sleeping aids such as Ambien, Xanax, Lunesta, or Benadryl work in a similar fashion, and the quality of your sleep takes a hit. Similarly, central nervous stimulants such as tobacco, caffeine, and exercise, throttle up your central nervous system, making the possibility of restful sleep less likely.

Jet lag is another reason for improper sleep patterns, though it is temporary. When you travel across continents, you don't just have to worry about packing and getting your tickets in order, but you also have to worry about the time differences. So if you land in London from New York at 7 p.m., it is just about lunchtime in New York! Besides wondering whether you will head out for lunch or dinner, your biological system that's still stuck in New York time might have to go to bed in a couple of hours!! So getting to bed and waking up at the right time will be a problem leading to sleep problems. Jet lag affects people to varying degrees, but it usually doesn't last for longer than two to three days.

THE HEALTH IMPACT OF POOR SLEEP

Poor sleep causes more problems than just being a little crabby in the morning. Here is a partial list of the negative repercussions of not getting the rest you need:

- increased risk of heart disease
- high blood pressure
- increased risk of obesity
- increased risk of type II diabetes
- impaired immune system
- cognitive impairment
- memory loss
- mood disorders and depression
- fatigue
- early-onset Alzheimer's disease or dementia
- accelerated aging
- tremors and musculoskeletal aches and pains

As you can see, sleep deprivation can and will pop your health balloon. The good news is that this problem can be prevented or fixed through some simple changes in lifestyle, and if necessary, a visit to a local physician who is well versed in integrative medicine.

DO YOU HAVE A SLEEPING PROBLEM?

How many of you remember the famous comedy routine of Jeff Foxworthy, "You might be a redneck if . . ." Let's apply this to the sleep problem.

YOU MIGHT BE SLEEP-DEPRIVED IF . . .

- You have problems falling asleep without the use of artificial tools such as sleeping pills, sedatives, or alcohol.
- You wake up multiple times throughout the night and have difficulty falling back to sleep because your mind is racing.
- You wake up tired and un-refreshed in the morning.
- You suffer from chronic fatigue throughout the day.
- You find yourself yawing during meetings.
- You can't keep your eyes open during important discussions or presentations.
- You require multiple naps daily just to get by.
- You are irritable or anxious and have difficulties concentrating or focusing on tasks.
- You're gaining weight and don't have enough "umph" to get out and exercise.
- Your overall state of health is declining, and you are always the first one in the family to catch the flu or the common cold.

Let's take a look at some of the causes of poor sleep patterns and what steps we can take to reclaim this precious gift.

SLEEP SOLUTIONS

Solutions in the quest for regular restful slumber consist of two general modalities: lifestyle changes and medical intervention.

Lifestyle changes: Although many of these recommendations may seem to be common sense, in the words of Will Rogers, "Common sense ain't so common." Try to incorporate these practices into your daily routine. You may be surprised by the fruit they bear.

- Most people need seven to nine hours of sleep each night. That's probably what you need, too. Try to go to sleep the same time every night, even on holidays, and try to get to bed before 11 p.m. The majority of your recovery and repair functions occur between the hours of 11 p.m. and 1 a.m. Not everyone needs nine hours of sleep every night, so it is important to find out your optimum time period and stick to it.

- Try to arrange an ideal sleep environment. That means comfortable bedding, a dark room, and no noise. Make sure that there is optimum ventilation and you are snug; improper ventilation or uneven beds tend to disturb sleep. Blaring TVs, barking dogs, and snoring spouses may require an investment in a good set of earplugs and eye pads (if it's not practical to remove these elements from your immediate surroundings).

- Prepare for sleep at least an hour before bedtime by winding down and avoiding intellectually stimulating activities such as reading a riveting murder mystery, surfing the Internet, debating the pros and cons of a fixed income tax, or worrying about all you have to do tomorrow. Consciously shut down your brain, and prep it to enter a restful state. Everything else can wait until tomorrow. Don't watch TV before bedtime, as you may fall asleep with the TV on, which will not result in a restful sleep.

- Although this may sound a bit New Age to some, try incorporating calming activities such as meditation, expressions of gratitude and appreciation, and prayer into your bedtime ritual.

- Try taking a hot bath or a sauna approximately one hour before bedtime.

- Avoid eating right before bedtime—especially sweets. A high-protein snack at least two hours before bedtime will hold you over until morning.

- Never, ever consume caffeinated products or alcohol within two hours of trying to go to sleep.
- Daily exercise is an important part of helping you sleep at night. However, try to avoid exercising within four hours of going to bed.
- If you find yourself staring at the ceiling, and you know that sleep isn't on the horizon, don't just lie there and toss and turn. Get up and go to another room, and do some light reading, or sit quietly listening to some restful music, then try again once a more relaxed state takes hold.
- Don't worry about not sleeping once you are in bed, as it increases anxiety, which in turn, will make it even more difficult to sleep.

MEDICAL INTERVENTION

If lifestyle changes are unsuccessful, you may have a physiologic reason for your sleeping problems. If your spouse tells you that you snore and sometimes stop breathing, you might have sleep apnea and should get that evaluated by a sleep specialist. Getting your sleep apnea treated isn't just good for you but also for the person who's sharing your room!

Medication side effects are a common cause of disrupted sleep. Insomnia is a side effect of many medications. Ask your physician for substitutes that don't trash your sleep.

Hormone imbalances are huge sleep "messer-uppers." Imbalances in estrogen, progesterone, testosterone, thyroid hormone, cortisol, melatonin, insulin, or human growth hormone are ALL well-known sleep killers and can wreak havoc on catching some shuteye. In our experience, this is the most common cause of disrupted sleep. As discussed elsewhere, hormonal balance can be easily attained.

Supplements such as L-tryptophan, melatonin, chamomile

tea, and phosphatidylserine are very powerful sleep aids, as they provide various calming effects on the central nervous system. Give these a try.

WHAT NOT TO DO IN YOUR QUEST FOR SLEEP

Today we live in a "pill for every ill" culture. On the surface, it's tempting to try the easy fix of a sedative or sleeping pill to help escort you to dreamland. Alcohol also falls into this category. Unfortunately, tons of research substantiates the fact that while these medications may help put you to sleep, they do a very poor job at keeping you asleep, and the sleep that you do get is of poor quality. It's relatively easy to find a physician to supply these medications for you, but avoid this temptation. There is a reason you are not sleeping well, and these medications are merely a shotgun attempt at addressing the symptom of sleeplessness while ignoring the cause. Be smart, diligent, and resourceful in uncovering the cause, and you will be rewarded for it. But if you do resort to these pills, remember that they may be okay once in a while, but in the long run, you could get addicted to them, or worse, might not be capable of sleeping on your own. A word of caution at this point: alcohol and pills should never be consumed together, as they can be a fatal combination and should be avoided at all costs.

Once you remove all of the roadblocks that disrupt sleep, it is important to maintain a sleep diary of everything that helps induce sleep. This could include soft lighting, listening to pleasant music, or even snuggling up with a pillow. As you continue to re-create the same situation every night, it becomes a habit, and the body falls into a natural sleep the minute you create the right environment.

To summarize, lack of sleep can have a profound effect on you psychologically, eventually damaging your health. The effects of sleep deprivation are cumulative and can creep up quite insidiously. If you aren't sleeping, find out why. Be selfish. Do everything you can to lay claim to seven to nine hours of sleep every night. This is your time—the time that you give yourself to be your best. If you are asked often why you look tired, then it's about time you set about ensuring that you get a good night's sleep. Seek medical attention from an integrative physician who can help tease out the causes if you aren't able to find it out yourself. You will be rewarded with optimized mental alertness and improved health that will have a huge impact on the experience of being alive and your quality of life, giving you the right start for the day.

CHAPTER 11

STEM CELLS, TELOMERES, GENETIC MANIPULATION . . . AND BEYOND

"*Stem cell therapy heals broken bones,*" "*Stem cells treat heart failure,*" "*Stem cells can be used to harvest tissues and organs,*" scream headlines every so often. Never has any research enjoyed such widespread attention like research on stem cells has.

Let's find out what these wonder cells actually are.

STEM CELLS

Stem cells have the ability to divide into many different types of cells during growth, much like an "all-rounder" in the game of baseball. The type of cells that a stem cell can develop into depends on its environment and the body's requirement for specific cell types. Though stem cells have the potential to transform into a wide variety of cells, once they transform into specific cells, they can never get back to their original form. This makes stem cells very special indeed. So where do these stem cells stem from? Let's get to the root of that!

STEM CELL ORIGINS

During early life, from the embryonic stage and during initial periods of growth, stem cells play an important role in differentiating into various types of cells to promote growth and development. Apart from this, stem cells are also present in certain organs and tissues, dividing whenever necessary to restore tissue for as long as the individual is alive.

Here are two unique features about stem cells that make them different from the other cells in your body:

- Stem cells can divide repeatedly by cell division even after prolonged periods of no activity.
- Stem cells can be induced to form specific cell types. This happens routinely in certain tissues like the gut and the bone marrow, while stem cells in the heart divide to form specific cells only under certain conditions. These cells divide rapidly, and it has been found that a starting population of stem cells in the laboratory can give rise to *millions* of cells. (Here's to population explosion!)

So where do you get these stem cells from? There are two different types of stem cells depending on where they are derived.

STEM CELL TYPES

Embryonic stem cells: These are derived from embryos and are the best type of stem cells, as they divide repeatedly even for a year under laboratory conditions! These cells come from embryos during the initial stages, when an embryo has only about eight cells in all. These embryonic cells develop to form the various tissues and organs in the body.

Embryonic stem cells that are used for research are obtained from embryos that are discarded during artificial reproduction techniques like In-vitro Fertilization (IVF), after informed consent from the mother. So these are merely cells that would never develop into a baby in any case.

These cells are extracted from the embryo and grown in culture dishes carefully. Scientists are diligently learning to understand how these cells are induced inside the human body to differentiate into specific cells. The introduction of certain chemicals or activating factors, when identified and included into the same dish as these stem cells, could give rise to specialized cells that can be used to treat a host of diseases including Parkinson's, diabetes, heart conditions, and Duchenne muscular dystrophy.

Of course, the use of embryonic stem cells entail huge moral and ethical objections for many. Their therapeutic use has been outlawed in the US and several other countries. That paints a dismal future for the advancement of stem cell science.

Adult stem cells: Yes! We have them, too! Adult stem cells are present in certain tissues and organs including the heart, peripheral blood, brain, bone marrow, testis, ovarian epithelium, liver, gut, teeth, skeletal muscle, and blood vessels. These stem cells, which are present in certain parts of the organs, will differentiate to form specific cells only under certain situations. Unfortunately, when scientists isolated these adult stem cells and tried culturing them in the laboratory, they didn't survive for as long as the embryonic stem cells did. These cells are still one up on the scientists, and intense research is on to try to understand the basis for this. The truth behind the numerous cell divisions that occur in embryonic stem cells but not in adult stem cells will help scientists understand the reason behind the uncontrolled cell division seen in cancer. Both embryonic and adult stem cells are difficult to acquire and may not be available in as large a quantity as is required for research. In order to overcome this, scientists use cultured induced pluripotent stem cells.

Induced pluripotent stem cells: These are adult cells that have been genetically re-programmed to express factors that are similar to stem cells. These cells are now used extensively for research.

Stem cells provide a great testing ground for pharmaceutical drugs. If you ever felt sorry for all the animals that were used to test drugs, you now have a chance to rejoice. Human stem cell cultures used in the laboratory are used for testing drugs, and the effects of these drugs on the cells will be similar to their effects on us, provided similar conditions are maintained. The cells are from us, after all!

If you are suffering from a broken heart, give stem cells a chance to mend it! Cardiovascular disease, which includes heart attacks and coronary heart disease, among others, is a leading cause of death. Lack of oxygen can lead to the death of cardiac muscle cells, which leads to a buildup of blood pressure inside the heart and the heart's eventual inability to pump sufficient amounts of blood. The strain on the heart can lead to a fatal heart attack and would require immediate surgery to prevent it. Researchers are studying the use of stem cells to replenish sup-plies of damaged heart tissue so that the heart is able to function as it normally does. Though this model has been successful in mice, it is yet to be determined in humans. Stem cells have been injected into the heart tissue during an open-heart surgery, and evidence has been collected about their effectiveness in build-ing new capillaries and heart tissues, though further conclusive evidence is still lacking.

Promises for new body tissue using stem cells doesn't just end with the heart but extends to the bone. Scientists from Saint

Luc University in Brussels have successfully treated eleven patients who either broke their bone or had some bone deficiency using stem cells injected into the site. What makes this study exciting is that the stem cells were not derived from bone marrow but were taken from fatty tissue. Adipose-derived stem cells, which are stem cells derived from fat tissue, are the current rage in science, as they are minimally invasive when compared with the other techniques. Shylock asked for "A pound of flesh" in *The Merchant of Venice;* well, that's all doctors might need to set your bone in order using adipocyte-derived stem cells.

The potential to use stem cells seem endless, as these cells can be effectively directed to replicate into different types of cells and introduced into the body to aid in repair of specific tissue. Many research studies are being carried out to identify procedures that will make this possible. Till then, we have to rely on the stem cells that do exist in our body to repair and renew our system periodically. As children, we have plenty of stem cells, but the amount of stem cells lessens as we age. Eventually, there is a complete lack of stem cells, ultimately leading to death. With man's yearning to stay young and healthy, stem cells offer a definite glimmer of hope. Like Bryan Adams' song, "18 Till I Die," there soon might be a future where stem cells are used to increase not just the number of years a person lives but also the quality of life in terms of restored tissues and organs.

Stem cells delay aging by aiding in the renewal of tissues in the body and helping the body manage "wear and tear." However, other indicators of aging are being scrutinized by the scientific population. One promising indicator of aging is the telomerase enzyme. Research on the telomerase enzyme netted three scientists the Nobel Prize in 2009.

TELOMERES

Telomeres are the tips of chromosomes which protect the end portions of the chromosome. These nucleotide sequences get shorter after every successive cell division, and their reduction is an indicator of old age or cancer: when telomeres are completely exhausted, cell death occurs. As the length of the telomeres get shorter, incidences of illnesses like heart disease increase. When a cell divides and there is chromosomal division, the chromosome may not divide till the end, resulting in the loss of important genetic information. To prevent this, telomeres are present at the tip; they are used during division and replenished by the enzyme telomerase reverse transcriptase. These fragments also prevent the tips of the chromosome from joining with other chromosome fragments and keep the chromosome from unraveling.

These seemingly unimportant sequences are like the fuse to a bomb; the minute the fuse runs out, time is up! With so much being said about telomeres, scientists have devised a test to determine the length of telomeres. This is to tell you where you stand biologically as far as aging is concerned, though physically it may be a different story! Telomere testing provides the length of your telomeres, and this can be used to determine your biological age. It can't determine how long you will live, but it can be used as a measure of the life that has gone by and the extent of telomere still available. Longer telomeres are indicative of fewer illnesses and a longer period of life.

A study published in the journal *The Lancet Oncology* has found that people who changed their lifestyle to a healthier one lived longer! Though this is no surprise, the study has found conclusive evidence that changes in food habits, exercise, and stress levels increase the length of telomeres over a period of time. In the study group, there was a 10 percent increase in the length of telomeres of individuals who underwent changes in their lifestyle, while there was a 3-percent decrease in telomere length in the control group (the group that did not undergo lifestyle changes).

"It sure feels good to be alive. Someday I'll be 18 going on 55." (That's Bryan Adams again crooning about staying young forever.) So is this the fountain of youth—the elixir that will help keep old age at bay? The increase in telomere length due to lifestyle changes sure seems to be a pause button in the race of life.

There is so much information in the chromosomal DNA, and if every cell in the body has the same DNA, ever wondered why a skin cell looks different from a brain cell? Well, it's all because of epigenetics.

EPIGENETICS

Epigenetics is the external control over our proteins' ability to read DNA. There are different types of epigenetic factors that exert control, and the most important is DNA methylation. Methyl groups are added to certain parts of the DNA sequence, preventing proteins from reading those parts.

Another example would be histones, or the proteins that bind certain regions of chromosomal DNA tightly together, denying the reading proteins access to those regions. It's pretty much like stapling a few pages of a book—you simply can't read those stapled pages!

It's interesting to note that these changes don't just exert their influence on the individual; they can also be inherited by the next generation. Generally, the sperms and the egg undergo certain modifications that reverse these epigenetic changes, but some of them are inherited by the embryo. This means that what a mother eats during pregnancy could actually influence the growth of the child! Food rich in methyl groups like folic acid influence the epigenetics of the unborn child, and children receiving inadequate amounts of folic acids or food rich in methyl groups could have lifelong changes to their epigenetic profile.

The influence of epigenetics is not only dependent upon the mother's diet but on the grandfather's, too! A study conducted in Sweden showed that grandfathers who ate small amounts of food between the ages of 9 and 12 had grandchildren who lived longer than the grandchildren of grandfathers who ate a lot during that time! Another bummer for eating too much! This was because overeating led to conditions like heart disease and diabetes, and this environmental information was transferred epigenetically to the grandchildren!

If you're now thinking, *"Big deal; everything the child has is inherited from the parents anyway, and epigenetics is no different,"* then here's some food for thought. The epigenetic changes that are inherited are those that are inherited without any actual change in the DNA sequence of the parents. Mothers who have diabetes during pregnancy (gestational diabetes) have high amounts of blood glucose in their body, resulting in epigenetic changes in the daughter's genetic information. This increases the chances of the daughter acquiring gestational diabetes during pregnancy significantly.

The changes that are part of epigenetics exert considerable influence on evolution, as epigenetics allow organisms to fit in with changes in the environment without actual changes to the DNA sequence. This is the difference between epigenetics and genetic mutation; the latter involves a change in the DNA sequence.

If life span and the risk of diseases are influenced by our forefathers and their diet, does the future seem completely bleak and out of your hands? Quite the contrary. After considerable analysis, scientists have discovered that diet during your adult life can reverse DNA methylation and other epigenetic changes. This means that we can eat our way out of our grandparents' genetic imprinting! With so much about our life and the illnesses that we might experience written in our genes, it does seem natural to have it "read" out so that we know exactly what we are in for. Genetic testing could pave the way for a more intelligent way of life.

GENETIC TESTING

Genetic testing is aimed at identifying single nucleotide polymorphisms in the DNA of an individual. Human DNA consists of four different types of nucleotides that are bonded together as specific pairs. Sometimes, one nucleotide is replaced with another, and this is called single nucleotide polymorphisms. Though these changes are not usually found within a gene, when they are present, they exert an influence and could lead to disease.

The significance of single nucleotide polymorphisms (called SNPs) is not only an indicator of impending disease, but is also an indicator of the individual's response to drugs, exercise, diet, risk factors for disease, and so on. Carrying out a genetic testing would be like seeing through a crystal ball into the future and identifying risk factors and situations that could be dangerous or harmful.

All of us have always been excited about knowing what lies in store for us. Finally, we have a choice of actually finding out. Genetic testing requires just a small sample of blood, after which the blood is screened for potential SNPs. The information gathered can then be used to lead a life that best avoids situations that could affect your longevity. For example, if an SNP lies in a major gene that could result in the development of diabetes, controlling your sugar intake could prevent the condition from occurring or becoming fatal.

To sum it all up, genetic testing is like being handed a card that lists everything that you can or cannot do to live a long, healthy, and fulfilling life.

ABOUT THE AUTHOR

Dr. Kevin Light attended Michigan State University, earning his Bachelor of Science degree in Biochemistry. He received an MBA from the University of Texas at Austin and attended medical school at Des Moines University. Dr. Light received his board certification in general surgery and served in several countries with the US Air Force for 7 years. He also attended the United States Air Force School of Aerospace Medicine and, as a Flight Surgeon, flew several missions in F-15 and F-16 fighter aircraft. Dr. Light was among the first surgical teams placed in Saudi Arabia during Operation Desert Storm and received two Air Force Commendation Medals.

Dr. Light practices Cosmetic Surgery and Integrative Medicine in Dallas, Texas. He is married with 4 children and a huge Rhodesian Ridgeback named Rusty. He is an avid skier and embraces international travel among his greatest passions.

FOR MORE INFORMATION

Algarté-Génin, M. O. Cussenot, P. Costa, et al. 2004. "Prevention of prostate cancer by androgens: experimental paradox or clinical reality?" *European Urology* 46: 285-95.

Almeida, O. P., B. B. Yeap, Graeme J. Hankey, et al. 2008. "Low free testosterone concentration as a potentially treatable cause of depressive symptoms in older men." *Archives of General Psychiatry* 65 (3): 283-89.

American Academy of Neurology. 2007. "HRT before Age 65 May Decrease Risk of Dementia and Alzheimer's Disease." Abstract S31.004. Presented at the American Academy of Neurology 59th Annual Meeting, April 28-May 5, Boston, Massachusetts.

Armario, A. 2006. "The hypothalamic-pituitary-adrenal axis: what can it tell us about stressors?" *CNS & Neurological Disorders - Drug Targets* 5 (5): 485-501.

Arnlöv, J., M. J. Pencina, S. Amin, et al. 2006. "Endogenous sex hormones and cardiovascular disease incidence in men." *Annals of Internal Medicine* 145 (3): 176-84.

Anagnostis, P., V. G. Athyros, K. Tziomalos, et al. 2009. "The pathogenic role of cortisol in the metabolic syndrome: a hypothesis." *Journal of Clinical Endocrinology & Metabolism* 94 (8): 2692-701.

Araujo, A. B., A. B. O'Donnell, D. J. Brambilla, et al. 2004. "Prevalence and incidence of androgen deficiency in middle-aged and older men: estimates from the Massachusetts male aging study." *Journal of Clinical Endocrinology & Metabolism* 89 (12): 5920-26.

Barrett-Connor, E., D. Goodman-Gruen, B. Patay, et al. 1999. "Endogenous sex hormones and cognitive function in older men." *Journal of Clinical Endocrinology & Metabolism* 84 (10): 3681-85.

Basaria, S., and A. S. Dobs. 1999. "Risks versus benefits of testosterone therapy in elderly men." *Drugs & Aging* 15 (2): 131-42.

Bassil, N., S. Alkaade, and J. E. Morely. 2009. "The benefits and risks of testosterone replacement therapy: a review." *Journal of Therapeutics and Clinical Risk Management* 5 (3): 427-48.

Bhasin, S. 2002. "The dose-dependent effects of testosterone on sexual function and on muscle mass and function." *Mayo Clinic Proceedings* 75 (January Suppl): S70-S75.

Bhasin, S., G. R. Cunningham, F. J. Hayes, et al. 2006. "Testosterone therapy in adult men with androgen deficiency syndromes: an endocrine society clinical practice guideline." *Journal of Clinical Endocrinology & Metabolism* 91 (6): 1995-2010.

Bhasin, S., W. Storer, N. Berman, et al. 1997. "Testosterone replacement increases fat-free mass and muscle size in hypogonadal men." *Journal of Clinical Endocrinology & Metabolism* 82 (2): 407-13.

Biondi, B., and L. Wartofsky. 2012. "Combination replacement of T4 and T3: toward personalized replacement of hypothyroidism." *Journal of Clinical Endocrinology & Metabolism* 97 (7): 2256-71. doi:10.1210/jc.2011-3399. Epub 16 May.

Björntorp, P. 1997. "Body fat distribution, insulin resistance, and metabolic diseases." *Nutrition* (9): 795-803.

Blackwell, J. 2004. "Evaluation and treatment of hyperthyroidism and hypothyroidism." *Journal of the American Academy of Nurse Practitioners* 16 (10): 422-25.

Boutcher, S. H. 2011. "High-intensity intermittent exercise and fat loss." 2011. *Journal of Obesity*: 868305. doi:10.1155/2011/868305. Epub 24 November 2010.

Brown, S. 2012. "Shock, terror and controversy: how the media reacted to the Women's Health Initiative." *Climacteric* 15: 275-80.

Buenevičius, R., Gintautas Kažanavičius, Rimas Žalinkevičius, et al. 1999. "Effects of thyroxine plus triiodothyronine as compared with hypothyroidism." *New England Journal of Medicine* 340 (6): 424-29.

Burris, A., Steven M. Banks, C. Sue Carter, et al. 1992. "A long term, prospective study of the physiologic and behavioral effects of hormone replacement in untreated hypogondal men." *Journal of Andrology* 13 (4): 297-304

Caminti, G. M. Volterrani, F. lellamo, et al. 2009. "Effect of long-acting testosterone treatment on functional exercise capacity, skeletal muscle performance, insulin resistance, and baroreflex sensitivity in elderly patients with chronic heart failure a double-bind, placebo-controlled, randomized study." *Journal of the American College of Cardiology* 54 (10): 919-27.

Centers for Disease Control and Prevention. "The benefits of physical activity" http://www.cdc.gov/physicalactivity/everyone/health/index.html. Accessed 5 July 2011.

Chrousos, G. P. 2000. "The role of stress and hypothalamic-pituitary-adrenal axis in the pathogenesis of the metabolic syndrome: neuroendocrine and target tissue-related causes." *International Journal of Obesity and Related Metabolic Disorders* 24: S50-S55.

Chrousos, G.P., and P. W. Gold. 1992. "The concept of stress and stress system disorders: overview of physical and behavioral homeostasis." *JAMA* 267 (9): 1244-52.

Clear, A. J., J. Miell, E. Heap, S. Sookdeo, et al. 2011. "Hypothalamo-pituitary-adrenal axis dysfunction in chronic fatigue syndrome and the effects of low-hydrocortisone therapy." *Journal of Clinical Endocrinology & Metabolism* 86 (8): 3545-54.

Cleveland Clinic. 2009. "Thyroid Disease." http://my.clevelandclinic.org/disorders/thyroid_cancer//hic_thyroid_cancer.aspx.

Clow, A., L. Thorn, P. Evans, and F. Hucklebridge. 2004. "The awakening cortisol response: methodological issues and significance." *Stress* 7 (1): 29-37.

Clyde, P. W., A. E. Harari, E. J. Getka, et al. 2003. "Combined levothyroxine plus liothyronine compared with levothyroxine alone in primary hypothyroidism: a randomized controlled trial." *JAMA* 290 (22): 2952-58.

Cooper, Kenneth H. 1997. *Can Stress Heal?* Nashville: Thomas Nelson Inc., p. 40. http://books.google.com/books?id=k75y6g5-aQAC&pg=PT40. Retrieved 19 October 2011.

Cornoldi, A., G. Caminiti, G. Marazzi, et al. 2009. "Effects of chronic testosterone administration on myocardial ischemia, lipid metabolism and insulin resistance in elderly male diabetic patients with coronary heart disease." *International Journal of Cardiology.* [Epub ahead of print 8 April.]

Danzi, S. and I. Klein. 2004. "Thyroid hormone and the cardiovascular system." *Minerva Endocrinologia* 29 (3): 139-50.

de Grey, Aubrey, and Michael Ray. 2008. *Ending Again: The Rejuvenation Breakthroughs That Could Reverse Human Aging in Our Lifetime.* Reprint, New York: St. Martin's Griffin.

De Mello Meirelles, C., P. S. C. Gomes. 2004. "Acute effects of resistance exercise on energy expenditure: revisiting the impact of the training variables" (pdf). *The Revista Brasileira de Medicina do Esporte* 10: 131–38. Retrieved 6 February2008.

Deroo, B. J., and K. S. Korach. 2006. "Estrogen receptors and human disease." *Journal of Clinical Investigation* 116 (3): 561-70.

Elmlinger, M.W., W. Kühnel, H. Wormstall, et al. 2005. "Reference intervals of testosterone, androstenedione and SHBG levels in healthy females and males from birth until old age." *Clinical Laboratory* 51 (11-12): 625-32.

El-Sakka, AI et al. 2005. "Prostatic specific antigen in patients with hypogonadism: effect of testosterone replacement." *Journal of Sexual Medicine* 2 (2): 235-40.

Escobar-Morreale, H. F., J. I. Botella-Carretero, M. Gómez-Bueno, et al. 2005. "Thyroid hormone replacement therapy in primary hypothyroidism: a randomized trial comparing L-thyroxine plus liothyronine with L-thyroxine alone." *Annals of Internal Medicine* 142 (6): 412-24.

Ewertz, M., L. Mellemkjaer, A. H. Poulson, et al. 2005. "Hormone use for menopausal symptoms and risk for breast cancer. A Danish cohort study." *British Journal of Cancer* 92 (7): 1293-97.

Fitzpatrick, L. A., C. Pace, and B. Wiita. 2000. "Comparison of regimens containing oral micronized progesterone or medroxyprogesterone acetate on quality of life in postmenopausal women: a cross-sectional survey." *Journal of Women's Health & Gender-Based Medicine* 9 (4): 381-87.

Formby, B., and T. S. Wiley. 1998. "Progesterone inhibits growth and induces apoptosis in breast cancer cells: inverse effects on Bcl-2 and p53." *Annals of Clinical and Laboratory Science* 28 (6): 360-69.

Fournier, A., F. Berrino, and F. Clavel-Chapelon. 2008. "Unequal risks for breast cancer associated with different hormone replacement therapies: results from the E3N cohort study." *Breast Cancer Research and Treat-*

ment 107 (1): 103-11. Epub 27 February 2007.

Freedman, D.M., A. C. Looker, S. C. Chang, et al. 2007. "Prospective study of serum vitamin D and cancer mortality in the United States." *Journal of the National Cancer Institute* 99 (21): 1594-602. Epub 30 October 2007.

Fries, E., J. Hesse, J. Hellhammer J, et al. 2005. "A new view on hypocortisolism." *Psychoneuroendocrinology* 10: 1010-16.

Galvao, D., and D. Taafee. 2004. "Single- vs. multiple-set resistance training: recent developments in the controversy." *Journal of Strength and Conditioning Research* 18: 660-67.

Genazzani, A. R., N. Pluchino, S. Luisi, et al. 2007. "Estrogen, cognition and female ageing". *Human Reproduction Update* 13 (2): 175-87.

Gibala, Martin J., Jonathan P. Little, Martin van Essen, et al. 2006. "Short-term sprint interval versus traditional endurance training: similar initial adaptations in human skeletal muscle and exercise performance" *Journal of Physiology* 575 (3): 901-11. doi:10.1113/jphysiol.2006.112094. Retrieved 23 July 2008.

Giovannucci, E., Y. Liu, B. W. Hollis, et al. 2008. "25-hydroxyvitamin D and risk of myocardial infarction in men: a prospective study." *Archives of Internal Medicine* 168 (11): 1174-80.

Goldstein, D. S., and I. J. Kopin. 2007. "Evolution concepts of stress" *Stress* 10 (2): 109-20.

Gould D. C., and R. S. Kirby. 2006. "Testosterone replacement therapy for late onset hypogonadism: what is the risk of inducing prostate cancer?" *Prostate Cancer and Prostatic Diseases* 9 (1): 14-18.

Hak, A. E., H. A. Pols, T. J. Visser, et al. 2002. "Subclinical hypothyroidism is an independent risk factor of atherosclerosis and myocardial infarction in elderly women: the Rotterdam Study." *Annals of Internal Medicine* 132 (4): 270-78.

Hall, G., and T. J. Phillips. 2005. "Estrogen and skin: the effects of estrogen, menopause, and hormone replacement therapy on the skin." *Journal of the American Academy of Dermatology* 53 (4): 555-68.

Harvard School of Public Health. "The nutrition source: simple steps to preventing diabetes." http://www.hsph.harvard.edu/nutritionsource/diabetes-full-story/.

Hayflick, Leonard. 1965. "The limited in vitro lifetime of human diploid cell strains." *Experimental Cell Research* 37 (3): 614-636.

Heim, C., U. Ehlert, and D. H. Hellhammer. 2000. "The potential role of hypocortisolism in the pathophysiology of stress-related bodily disorders." *Psychoneuroendocrinology* 25 (1): 1-35.

Hoffman, M. A. 2002. "Is low serum free testosterone a marker for high grade prostate cancer?" *Journal of Urology* 163 (3): 824-27.

Hogervorst, E., S. Bandelow, M. Combrinck, , et al. 2004. "Low free testosterone is an independent risk factor for Alzheimer's disease." *Experimental Gerontology* 39 (11-12): 1633-39.

Holloszy, J. O., and E. F. Coyle. 1984. "Adaptations of skeletal muscle to endurance exercise and their metabolic consequences." *Journal of Applied Physiology: Respiratory, Environmental and Exercise Physiology* 56: 831-38.

Holtorf, K. 2008. "Diagnosis and treatment of hypothalamic-pituitary-adrenal (hpa) axis dysfunction in patients with chronic fatigue syndrome (CFS) and fibromyalgia (FM)." *Journal of Chronic Fatigue Syndrome* 14 (3): 1-14.

Holtorf, K. 2009. "The bioidentical hormone debate: are bioidentical hormones (estradiol, estriol, and progesterone) safer or more efficacious than commonly used synthetic versions in hormone replacement therapy?" *Postgraduate Medicine* 121 (1): 73-85.

"How to Read a Nutritional Label." WebMD. http://www.webmd.com/food-recipes/features/how-read-nutrition-label.

Hu, Frank B., JoAnn E. Manson, Mier J. Stampfer, et al. 2001. "Diet, lifestyle, and the risk for type 2 diabetes mellitus in women." *New England Journal of Medicine* 345: 790-97.

Ikehara, S., H. Iso, and C. Date, et al. 2009. "Association of sleep duration with mortality from cardiovascular disease and other causes for Japanese men and women: the JACC study." *Sleep* 32 (3): 259-301.

Jackson, G., N. Boon, I. Eardley, et al. 2010. "Erectile dysfunction and coronary and heart disease prediction: evidence-based guidance and consensus." *International Journal of Clinical Practice* 64 (7): 848-57.

Joffe, R. T., M. Brimacombe, A. J. Levitt, et al. 2007. "Treatment of clinical hypothyroidism with thyroxine and triiodothyronine; a literature review and meta-analysis." *Psychosomatics* 48 (5): 379-84.

Kabat, G. C., E. S. O'Leary, M. D. Gammon, et al. 2006. "Estrogen metabolism and breast cancer." *Epidemiology* 17 (1): 80-88.

Kenny, A. M., A. Kleppinger, K. Annis, et al. 2010. "Effects of transdermal testosterone on bone and muscle in older men with low bioavailable testosterone levels, low bone mass, and physical frailty." *Journal of the American Geriatrics Society* 58 (6): 1134-43.

Kim J., S. Y. Lim, A. Shin, et al. 2009. "Fatty fish and omega-3 fatty acid intakes decrease the breast cancer risk: a case-control study." *BMC Cancer* 9: 216.

Krotkiewski, M. 2002. "Thyroid hormones in the pathogenesis and treatment of obesity." *European Journal of Pharmacology* 440 (2-3): 85-98.

Kudielka, B. M., D. S. Hellhammer, and S. Wüst. 2009. "Why do we respond so differently? Reviewing determinants of human salivary cortisol responses to challenge." *Psychoneuroendocrinology* 34: 2-18.

Kudielka, B. M., N. C. Schommaker, D. H. Hellhammer, et al. 2004. "Acute HPA axis responses, heart rate and mood changes to psychosocial stress (TSST) in humans at different times of day." *Psychoneuroendocrinology* 8: 983-92.

Laurin, D., R. Verreault, J. Lindsay, et al. 2001. "Physical activity and risk of cognitive impairment and dementia in elderly persons." *Archives of Neurology* 58: 498-504.

Laursen, P. B., and D. G. Jenkins. 2002. "The scientific basis for high-intensity interval training: optimising training programmes and maximising performance in highly trained endurance athletes." *Sports Medicine* 32 (1): 53-73.

Leitzmann, M. F., E. A. Platz, Stampfer, M. J., et al. 2004. "Ejaculation frequency and subsequent risk of prostate cancer." *JAMA* 291 (13): 1578-86.

Iervasi G., A. Pingitore, P. Landi, et al. 2003. "Low T3-syndrome; a strong prognostic predictor of death in patients with heart disease." *Circulation* 107 (5): 708-13.

L'hermite, M., T. Simoncini, S. Fuller, et al. 2008. "Could transdermal estradiol + progesterone be a safer postmenopausal HRT? A review." *Maturitas* 60, no 3-4:185-201. Epub 5 September.

Little, Jonathan P., Adeel S. Safdar, Geoffrey P. Wilkin, et al. 2009. "A practical model of low-volume high-intensity interval training induces mitochondrial biogenesis in human skeletal muscle: potential mechanisms." *Journal of Physiology* 588 (Pt. 6): 1011–22. doi:10.1113/jphysiol.2009.181743.

Maggio, M., S. Basaria, G. P. Ceda, et al. 2005. "The relationship between testosterone and molecular markers of inflammation in older men." *Journal of Endocrinological Investigation* 28 (11 Suppl Proceedings): 116-19.

Mahmud, K. 2009. "Natural hormone therapy for menopause." *Gynecological Endocrinology* 19: 1-5. [Epub ahead of print.]

McArdle, William D., Frank I. Katch, and Victor L. Katch. 2006. *Essentials of Exercise Physiology*. Philadelphia: Lippincott Williams & Wilkins,p. 204. http://books.google.com/books?id=L4aZIDbmV3oC&pg=PA204. Retrieved 13 October 2011.

McAuley, E., A. Kramer, and S. Colombe. 2004. "Cardiovascular fitness and neurocognitive function in older adults: A brief review." *Brain, Behavior and Immunity* 18 (3): 214-20.

McEwen, B. 1998. "Protective and Damaging Effects of Stress Mediators." *New England Journal of Medicine* 338 (3): 171-77.

------. 1998. "Stress, adaptation and disease. Allostasis and allostatic load." *Annals of the New York Academy of Sciences* 840: 33-44.

------. 2008. "Central effects of stress hormones in health and disease: understanding the protective and damaging effects of stress mediators." *European Journal of Pharmacology* 583: 174-85.

McEwen, B. S., and P. J. Gianaros. 2010. "Central role of the brain in stress and adaptation: links to socioeconomic status, health and disease." *Annals of the New York Academy of Sciences* 1186: 190-222.

Miller, H. "Response to 'The bioidentical hormone debate: are bioidentical hormones (estradiol, estriol, and progesterone) safer or more effica-cious than commonly used synthetic versions in hormone replacement therapy?'" *Postgraduate Medicine* 121 (4): 172.

Minaker, K. L. 2007. "Common Clinical Sequelae of Aging." In *Goldman's Cecil Medicine,* 23rd edition, by Lee Goldman and Dennis Ausiello, chap-ter 24. Philadelphia: Elsevier/Saunders.

Morales, A. 2002. "Androgen replacement therapy and prostate safety." *European Urology* 41 (2): 113-20.

Morgentaler, A. 2006. "A Testosterone and Prostate Cancer: A Historical Perspective on a Modern Myth." *European Urology* 50 (5): 935-39. Epub 27 July 2006.

National Library of Medicine, National Institutes of Health. 2012. "Aging changes in hormone production." http://www.nlm.nih.gov/medineplus/ency/article/004000.htm.

National Sleep Foundation. 2001. "Sleep in America" Poll. National Sleep Foundation, Washington, DC.

Norwegian University of Science and Technology. 2011. "Feed your genes." http://www.ntnu.edu/news/feed-your-genes.

Park, A. 2008. "Lack of Sleep Linked to Heart Problems." http://www.Time.com. December 23.

Perry, C. G., G. J. Heigenhauser, A. Bonen, et al. 2008. "High-intensity aerobic interval training increases fat and carbohydrate metabolic capac-ities in human skeletal muscle." *Applied Physiology, Nutrition, and Metab-olism* 33 (6): 1112-23.

Peterson, D. M. "Overview of the benefits and risks of exercise." http://www.uptodate.com/home/index.html. Accessed 6 June 2011.

Pines, A., D. W. Sturdee, and A. H. MacLennan. 2012. "Quality of life and the role of menopausal therapy." *Climacteric* 15: 213-16.

Plowman, Sharon A., and Denise L. Smith. 2007. *Exercise Physiology for Health, Fitness, and Performance.* Philadelphia: Lippincott Williams & Wilkins, p. 61. Retrieved 13 October 2011.

Purbrick, B., K. Stranks, C. Sum, et al. 2012. "Future long-term trials of postmenopausal hormone replacement therapy-what is possible and what is the optimal protocol and regimen?" *Climacteric* 15: 288-93.

Reeves, W. C., F. Jones, E. Maloney, et al. 2007. "Prevalence of chronic fatigue syndrome in metropolitan, urban and rural Georgia." *Population Health Metrics* 5: 5.

Reynaud, J. P. 2009. "Testosterone deficiency syndrome: treatment and cancer risk." *Journal of Steroid Biochemistry and Molecular Biology* 114 (1-2): 96-105.

Rupp, H., D. Wagner, T. Rupp, et al. 2004. "Risk stratification by the "EPA+DHA level" and the "EPA /AA ratio" focus on anti-inflammatory and antiarrhythmogenic effects of long chain omega-3 fatty acids". *Herz* 29 (7): 673-85.

Salpeter, S. R., J. M. E. Walsh, T. M. Ormiston, et al. 2006. Meta-analysis: effect of hormone-replacement therapy on components of the metabolic syndrome in postmenopausal women. *Diabetes, Obesity and Metabolism* 8: 538–54.

Schuder, S. E. 2006. "Stress-induced hypocortisolemia diagnosed as psychiatric disorders responsive to hydrocortisone replacement." *Annals of the New York Academy of Sciences* 1507: 466-478.

Schumacher, M., R. Guennoun, A. Ghoumari, et al. 2007. "Novel perspectives for progesterone in hormone replacement therapy, with special reference to the nervous system." *Endocrine Reviews* 28 (4): 387-439. Epub 12 April 2007.

Schwartz, E. T., and K. Holtorf. 2008. "Hormones in wellness and disease prevention: common practices, current state of the evidence, and questions for the future." *Primary Care* 35 (4): 669-705.

Seidman, S. N., G. Orr, G. Raviv, et al. 2009. "Effects of testosterone replacement in middle-aged men with dysthymia: a randomized, placebo-controlled clinical trial." *Journal of Clinical Psychopharmacology* 29 (3): 216-21.

Shores, M. M., D. R. Kivlahan, T. I. Sadak, et al. 2009. "A randomized, double-blind, placebo-controlled study of testosterone treatment in hypogonadal older men with subthreshold depression (dysthymia or minor depression)." *Journal of Clinical Psychiatry* 70 (7): 1009-16.

Simon, James. A. "Introduction: An overview of progesterone and progestins." *The Journal of Family Practice* (2 Suppl): S3-S5. Simon notes, "Clinicians have numerous options in selecting a progestogen for the individual patient. The specific properties of progesterone or synthetic progestins may result in differing side-effect profiles for individual patients. Route of administration also offers differing systemic or local effects that should be considered for some uses and specific patients. Differences exist among the exogenous progestogens, which include both natural progesterone and synthetic and semi-synthetic progestins, drugs which are "structurally related—but are not identical—to either progesterone or testosterone . . . Additionally, studies often do not evaluate the effects of progestogens on specific organs or compare the side-effect profiles of individual agents. These characteristics constitute an important, although rarely discussed, aspect of the differences among progestogens."

Simpoulos, A. P. 2002. "Omega fatty acids in inflammation and autoimmune diseases." *Journal of the American College of Nutrition* 21 (6): 495-505.

Simpson, N., and D. F. Dinges. 2007. "Sleep and inflammation." *Nutrition Reviews* 65 (12 Pt. 2): S244-52.

Smith, G. D., Y. Ben-Shlomo, A. Beswick, et al. 2005. "Cortisol, testosterone and coronary heart disease: prospective evidence from the Caerphilly study." *Circulation* 112 (3): 332-40.

Snyder, P. J., H. Peachey, J. A. Berlin, et al. 2000. "Effects of testosterone replacement in hypogonadal men." *Journal of Clinical Endocrinology & Metabolism.* 85 (8): 2670-77.

Sorensen, Janelle, Pooja Mott, and Brian Yablon. 2009. "Not So Sweet: Missing Mercury and High Fructose Corn Syrup." Institute of Agriculture and Trade Policy (IATP). http://www.iatp.org/files/421_2_105091.pdf. Published 26 January.

Stansfield C. A., R. Fuhrer, M. J. Shipley, et al. 2002. "Psychological distress as a risk factor for coronary in the Whitehall II Study." *International Journal of Epidemiology* 31 (1): 248-55.

Stattin, P. et al. 2004. "High levels of circulating testosterone are not associated with increased prostate cancer risk: a pooled prospective study." *International Journal of Cancer* 108 (3): 418-24.

Stellato, R. K., H. A. Feldman, O. Hamdy, et al. 2000. "Testosterone, sex hormone-binding globulin, and the development of type 2 diabetes in middle-aged men: prospective results from the Massachusetts male aging study." *Diabetes Care* 23 (4): 490-94.

Tabata I., K. Nishimura, M. Kouzaki, et al. 1996. "Effects of moderate-intensity endurance and high-intensity intermittent training on anaerobic capacity and VO2 max." *Medicine & Science in Sports & Exercise* 28 (10): 1327-30. doi:10.1097/00005768-199610000-00018.

"The Dirty Dozen Foods Additives You Really Need to be Aware of." *Sixwise.com.* Six Wise Newsletter 5 April 2006.

Tornhage, C. J. 2009. "Salivary cortisol for assessment of hypothalmic-pituitary-adrenal axis function." *Nueroimmunomodulation* 16 (5): 284-89.

Trapp E. G., D. J. Chisholm, J. Freund, et al. 2008. "The effects of high-intensity intermittent exercise training on fat loss and fasting insulin levels of young women." *International Journal of Obesity* 32 (4): 684-91. doi:10.1038/sj.ijo.0803781.

Traviscon, T. G., A. B. Araujo, V. Kupelian, et al. 2007. "The relative contributions of aging, health, and lifestyle factors to serum testosterone decline in men." *Journal of Clinical Endocrinology & Metabolism* 92, no. 2: 549-55. Epub 5 December 2006.

Van Gorp, T., and P. Neven. 2002. "Endometrial safety of hormone replacement therapy: review of literature." *Maturitas* 42 (2): 93-104.

Van Houdenhove, B., U. Egle, and P. Luyten. 2005. "The rate of life stress in fibromyalgia." *Current Rheumatology Reports* 7 (5): 365-70.

von Schacky, Clemens. 2003. "A review of omega-3 ethyl esters for cardiovascular prevention and treatment of increased blood triglyceride levels." *Journal of Vascular Health and Risk Management* 2 (3): 251-61.

Walsh, J. P., L. Shiels, E. M. Lim, et al. "Combined thyroxine/liothyronine treatment does not improve well-being, quality of life, or cognitive function compared to thyroxine alone: a randomized controlled trial in patients with primary hypothyroidism." *Journal of Clinical Endocrinology & Metabolism* 88: 4543-50.

Wang, C., R. S. Swerdloff, A. Iranmanesh, et al. 2000. "Transdermal testosterone gel improves sexual function, mood, muscle strength, and body composition parameters in hypogonadal men." *Journal of Clinical Endo-*

crinology & Metabolism 85 (8): 2839-53.

Wartofsky, L., and R. A. Dickey. 2005. "The evidence for a narrower thyrotropin reference range is compelling." Journal of Clinical Endocrinology & Metabolism 90 (9): 5483-88.

Wartofsky, L., D. Van Nostrand, and K. D. Burman. 2006. "Overt and 'subclinical' hypothyroidism in women." Obstetrical & Gynecological Survey 6 (8): 535-42.

Yeap, B. B. 2009. "Are declining testosterone levels a major risk factor for ill-health in aging men?" International Journal of Impotence Research 21 (1): 24-36.

------. 2009. "Testosterone and ill-health in aging men." Nature Clinical Practice Endocrinology & Metabolism 5 (2): 113-21.

Yeap, B. B., S. A. Chubb, Z. Hyde, et al. 2009. "Lower serum testosterone is independently associated with insulin resistance in non-diabetic older men: the Health in Men Study." European Journal of Endocrinology 161 (4): 591-98. doi:10.1530/EJE-09-0348. Epub 6 August.

Yeap, B. B., Z. Hyde, O. P. Almeida, et al. 2009, "Lower testosterone levels predict incident stroke and transient ischemic attack in older men." Journal of Clinical Endocrinology & Metabolism 94 (7): 2353-59. doi:10.1210/jc.2008-2416. Epub 7 April.

NOTES:

NOTES:

NOTES:

NOTES:

NOTES: